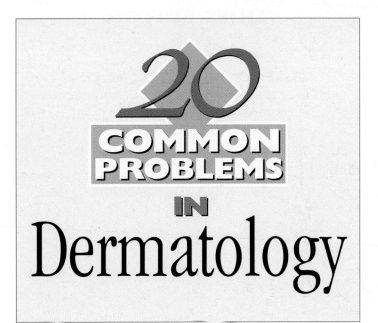

20 COMMON PROBLEMS IN Dermatology

Test 2→
Ch 8-16 (but not Ch9)

SERIES EDITOR

BARRY D. WEISS, M.D.
Professor of Clinical Family and Community Medicine
University of Arizona College of Medicine
Tucson, Arizona

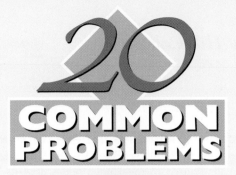

20 COMMON PROBLEMS IN Dermatology

ALAN B. FLEISCHER, JR., M.D.

Associate Professor of Dermatology
Westwood-Squibb Center for Dermatology Research and the Department of Dermatology
Wake Forest University School of Medicine
Winston-Salem, NC

STEVEN R. FELDMAN, M.D., PH.D.

Associate Professor of Dermatology
Westwood-Squibb Center for Dermatology Research and the Department of Dermatology
Wake Forest University School of Medicine
Winston-Salem, NC

AARON S. KATZ, M.D.

Private Practice
Spartanburg, SC

BETH D. CLAYTON, M.D.

Private Practice
Greenville, SC

McGraw-Hill

Health Professions Division

New York   St. Louis   San Francisco   Auckland   Bogotá   Caracas   Lisbon   London   Madrid
Mexico City   Milan   Montreal   New Delhi   San Juan   Singapore   Sydney   Tokyo   Toronto

McGraw-Hill College

A Division of The **McGraw·Hill** *Companies*

20 COMMON PROBLEMS IN DERMATOLOGY

Copyright © 2000 by The McGraw-Hill Companies, Inc. All rights reserved. Printed in the United States of America. Except as permitted under the United States Copyright Act of 1976, no part of this publication may be reproduced or distributed in any form or by any means, or stored in a data base or retrieval system, without the prior written permission of the publisher.

1234567890 1IMP 1IMP 99

ISBN 0-07-022067-0

This book was set in Garamond by York Graphic Services, Inc.
The editors were Joseph Hefta, Susan R. Noujaim, and Karen G. Edmonson;
The production supervisor was Richard Ruzycka
The text was designed by Marsha Cohen/Parallelogram
The index was prepared by Barbara Littlewood.
Printed and bound by Imago (U.S.A.), Inc., in Hong Kong.

This book is printed on acid-free paper.

Library of Congress Cataloging-in-Publication Data

20 common problems in dermatology / editors, Alan Fleischer, Jr. . . .
   [et al.].
     p. cm
   Includes bibliographical references and index.
   ISBN 0-07-022067-0
   1. Skin—Diseases Handbooks, manuals, etc. 2. Dermatology
Handbooks, manuals, etc. I. Fleischer, Alan B. II. Title: Twenty
common problems in dermatolory
   [DNLM: 1. Skin Diseases—diagnosis. 2. Skin Diseases—therapy.
WR 140 Z999 2000]
RL74.A14 2000
616.5—dc21
DNLM/DLC
for Library of Congress   99-32475
                      CIP

Contents

Part

3

Skin Growths and Tumors   191

Part

4

Miscellaneous Skin Diseases   247

Preface

Thousands of dermatologic diseases and conditions have been named and newly recognized conditions appear in the medical literature on a daily basis yet the most common skin disorders account for the overwhelming majority of patient visits to primary care providers and dermatologists. If one knows the 20 common problems described in this book well, one knows a great deal.

What are the common skin problems? The National Ambulatory Medical Care Survey provides representative data on the outpatient practice of medicine in the United States that we have used to determine the 20 most common skin disorders seen in primary care. These "20 common problems" account for 80 percent of the visits to primary care physicians for the treatment of skin disease.[1,2] Moreover, the treatment principles described for these conditions also apply to many of the remaining conditions.

Why study the common skin conditions? These conditions account for 5 to 10 percent of all visits to primary care physicians. They represent a challenge for many clinicians, as patients with the most common skin disorders are more likely to require referral than are patients with other medical disorders.[3] Seemingly "simple" skin disorders are not straightforward to manage. For instance, effectively managing acne requires one to understand patients' expectations about care, deal with an armamentarium of therapeutic agents that vastly exceeds the numbers of agents used to manage diabetes mellitus, and follow patients over time to monitor effectiveness and toxicity. Treatment of skin cancer goes beyond the diagnostic expertise of recognizing skin cancers and the technical expertise of removing them. The process of care involves weighing the benefits and risks of various surgical options, cosmetic concerns, cost-containment strategies, medical contraindications, and patient preferences.

Dermatologic problems cause severe morbidity, disfigurement, and disability. Accordingly, patients perceive them to be extraordinarily important for physicians to recognize and treat appropriately. All clinicians should realize that skin diseases are more than just skin deep; thus, skin diseases have an impact on health-related quality of life. For example, psoriasis patients report a reduction in physical and mental functioning comparable to that seen in patients with cancer, arthritis, hypertension, heart disease, diabetes and depression.[4] This book provides practical advice on the diagnosis and management of these common skin disorders. We have included selected treatment algorithms and referral guidelines to assist in the management of these patients. Patient care is optimized when clinicians understand and respect their individual limitations and have collegial relationships with their dermatologist colleagues.

References

1. Fleischer AB Jr, Feldman SR, McConnell RC: The most common skin problems seen by family practitioners, 1990–1994. *Fam Med* 29:648, 1997.

2. Feldman SR, Fleischer AB Jr, McConnell RC: Most common dermatologic problems identified by internists, 1990–1994. *Arch Intern Med* 158:726, 1998..

3. Feldman SR, Fleischer AB Jr, Chen JG: The gatekeeper model is inefficient for the delivery of dermatologic services. *J Am Acad Dermatol* 40:426, 1999.

4. Rapp SP, Exum ML, Feldman SR, et al: the Impact of psoriasis on health-related quality of life is similar to that of other medical diseases. *J Am Acad Dermatol,* in press.

This text is dedicated to one of the authors, Steve Feldman. Without his keen insight, boundless enthusiasm, genuine friendship, and true scholarship, this book could not have been produced.

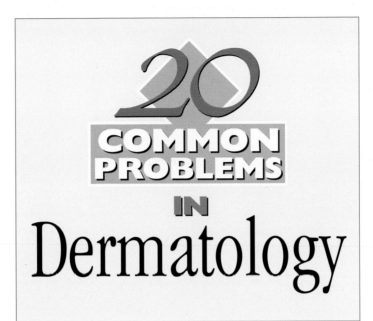

20 COMMON PROBLEMS IN Dermatology

Inflammatory
Skin Diseases

Acne Vulgaris

Background

Acne vulgaris is a common self-limited disease that presents with a variety of lesions, including open and closed comedones, pustules, nodules, and inflammatory papules. Although nearly universal in the teenage years, acne may continue until the third through fifth decades. It is a condition that has been associated with negative self esteem, and treatment may not only improve self confidence but prevent scarring.

Risk Factors

Acne can begin at any age, but hormonal influences make it more common in the middle to late teenage years. There is a slight predominance in men, who also commonly have more severe involvement. Despite the disparate sex ratio, more women seek treatment. There may be a familial influence, especially in severe cases. The incidence is equal in all races.

Patients who have recently received systemic corticosteroidal agents may develop severe acne rapidly. Similarly, those who take anabolic steroids to build muscle mass may develop severe acne suddenly. Other medications have a tendency to exacerbate acne, including lithium and birth control agents such as medroxyprogesterone (Depo-Provera) and oral contraceptive agents.

The use of specific cosmetic agents, ranging from abrasive cleansers to foundations and moisturizing creams, may exacerbate acne on an individual and idiosyncratic basis. Unfortunately, no cosmetics or toiletries are guaranteed to be free of acnegenicity.

Patients often focus on foods as potent agents that may exacerbate acne vulgaris. However, there is no convincing evidence that dietary factors play a role in producing or exacerbating acne. Many women, for instance, have perimenstrual acne flares that they attribute to diet rather than to their changing hormonal milieu. A practical approach is to allow patients to eat any foods they do not believe make their acne worse.

Pathophysiology

Acne vulgaris is a chronic disease of the pilosebaceous unit. The primary alteration is desquamation of follicular corneocytes into the sebaceous follicle ducts, forming a plug. When present for a prolonged period, the plug can be seen clinically as a comedone (Figs. 1-1 and 1-2). Acne patients tend to have larger sebaceous glands and produce more sebum than do persons without acne. However, patients with very dry skin also may have a great deal of acne activity. Nevertheless, the free fatty acid portion of sebum may be a contributing cause of inflammation. The anaerobic diphtheroid *Propionibacterium acnes*, which is found in hair follicles, is important in inducing inflammation through chemotactic factors and host response.

Androgenic stimulation is important in both men and women because it drives sebaceous gland secretion. Other hormonal influences also may play a role; women often have exacerbations of acne activity in the perimenstrual period. Emotional stressors appear to play a role in acute acne exacerbations but not in chronic acne vulgaris.

History

Acne vulgaris is a chronic, intermittent disease which may persist long past the teenage years; it is not unusual to find acne activity in the third and fourth decades of life. Acne becomes rare in women after menopause but can persist into the sixth decade in some men. Acne lesions are usually asymptomatic, although the nodules can be painful. Occasionally, patients complain of itching in the acne lesions. More darkly pigmented patients may be more bothered by the postinflammatory hyperpigmentation than by the acneiform lesions.

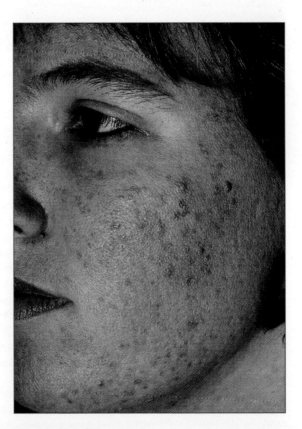

Figure 1-1

Multiple inflammatory papules and comedones.

Figure 1-2

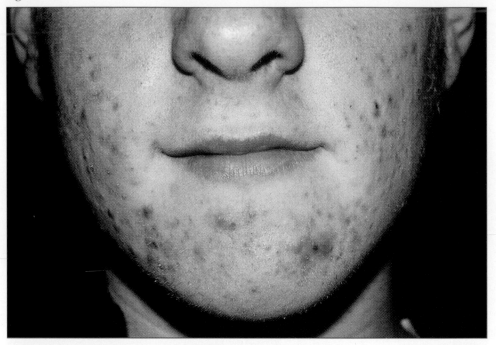

Inflammatory papules and nodules with scarring.

Physical Examination

The primary sites of acne are the face, chest, shoulders, and back. Lesions consist of open comedones (whiteheads), closed comedones (blackheads), pustules, erythematous papules, and deeper nodules (cysts) (Figs. 1-3 through 1-8). One type of lesion may predominate, but a variety often are found in various phases of development. When eruptive inflammatory acne lesions are all in the same stage of development, a common cause is systemic corticosteroid administration in the preceding few weeks or months.

The severity can range from mild acne with only comedones to severe nodular acne with a marked potential for disfiguring scars. Patients with severe acne often do not appreciate the severity of the scarring because they have not seen their noninflamed faces in months to years. The scarring process also may embed follicular epithelium remnants in the dermis, leading to the development of epidermoid cysts.

A common form of acne—acne excoriée—is caused by picking of facial lesions or perceived facial lesions. The physical examination shows excoriated, crusted lesions with few, if any, primary comedones or inflammatory lesions.

Figure 1-3

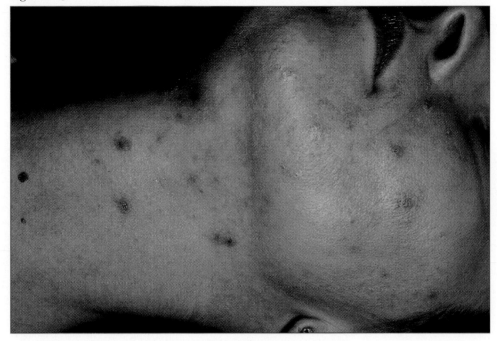

Inflammatory papules with evidence of picking behavior.

Laboratory Evaluation

Acne vulgaris is diagnosed clinically, and laboratory studies usually are not useful. The combination of severe acne with hirsutism, irregular menses, and obesity in women may warrant a gynecologic endocrinology evaluation for polycystic ovary syndrome. This evaluation may include obtaining serum levels of total and free plasma testosterone and dihydroepiandrosterone sulfate (DHEAS).

Complications

The major sequela of acne is scarring, which usually results from nodulocystic lesions. Therapy for scarring usually requires surgical procedures such as collagen injection, dermabrasion, and excision. Gram-negative folliculitis may develop in

Figure 1-4

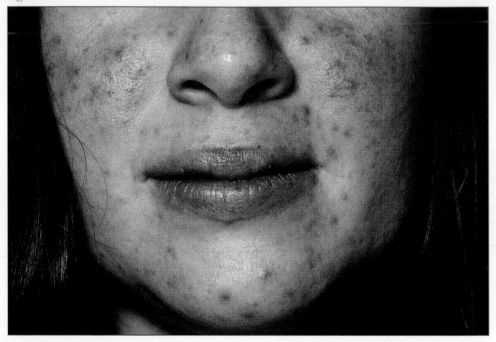

Inflammatory papules.

patients who receive prolonged antibiotic therapy and is heralded by the sudden flare of pustules or nodules in a patient who has been improving.

Psychological factors may play a significant role in acne management. In an appearance-oriented culture, acne has been demonstrated to lower the health-related quality of life. Acne can predispose a patient to low self-esteem, social phobias, and depression. In extreme cases, when acne is associated with depression, it can lead to self-destructive behavior and suicide. Since acne is not confined to the teenage years and because many physicians regard it as trivial, patients can be affected adversely by the social and psychological effects it engenders.

Treatment

Therapy for acne vulgaris varies according to the types of lesions present as well as the severity. Additionally, patient expectation varies remarkably between affected individuals. Some patients with "minor" disease may go to extraordinary lengths to treat acne, whereas some with severe disease may choose minimal or no treatment. In general, acne that is primarily comedonal responds best to topical retinoid agents and acid products (Fig. 1-9). Inflammatory lesions such as papules and pustules require either topical antibiotic agents when minor or oral antibiotic agents when major. The mechanism of action of antibiotics for acne is not perfectly clear as these agents are not only antimicrobial: They diminish inflammatory cell chemotaxis, modify the complement pathways, and inhibit the polymorphonuclear leukocyte chemotactic factor and lipase production in *P. acnes*.

Combinations of comedolytic agents and antibiotic agents are beneficial for the majority of these patients. Acne that is more severe, unresponsive to several systemic antibiotics, and characterized by mainly nodular lesions may be a good candidate for systemic isotretinoin therapy. Another useful approach for the acute treatment of painful nodules is intralesional corticosteroid injection.

If patients spend a great deal of time picking their skin, decreasing their fixation is an essential component of therapy. This may be accomplished with behavioral interventions, intensive medical therapy for the acne, or in extreme cases, treatment for obsessive-compulsive traits or disease.

Topical Therapies

RETINOID AGENTS

TRETINOIN Agents with tretinoin (retinoic acid; Retin A, Avita) are comedolytic and often are used in conjunction with antibacterial agents. They may produce signif-

Figure 1-5

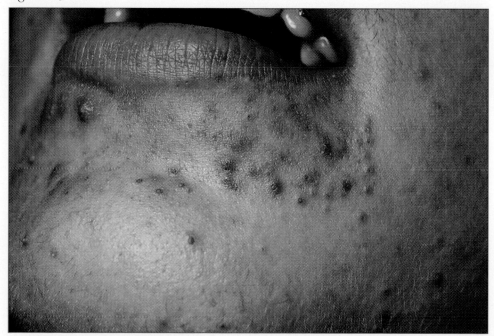

Predominantly comedonal acne of the chin.

icant erythema and dryness as a side effect. They are best used once nightly and applied sparingly. Mild photosensitivity may occur initially, but after 2 weeks of use there is no increased sun sensitivity. Tretinoin is available in a wide variety of vehicles and concentrations. Retin A Micro may have fewer side effects than does the standard gel because of its slow-release formula.

We generally start patients on Retin A 0.025% cream unless they have oily skin. If this is well tolerated, patients can increase the potency to the 0.05 or 0.1% strengths. Patients with oily skin may tolerate higher initial cream concentrations, or the gel may be used. Avita is available only in one concentration of cream or gel. Patients should be cautioned that tretinoin may initially exacerbate acne, although improvement will follow. Some patients may require 1 to 2 months of therapy to become accustomed to this agent. We counsel patients to begin with small amounts of the drug and gradually increase the quantity as the skin becomes tolerant. Tretinoin should not be applied at the same time benzoyl peroxide products are applied, as it may not retain its chemical stability.

ADAPALENE   Adapalene (Differin) is another retinoid agent that is available for topical acne use. Its efficacy is similar to or slightly better than that of Retin A 0.025% gel, and it is available in either gel or solution. Like tretinoin products, adapalene is comedolytic and often is used in conjunction with antibacterial agents. It produces significant erythema and dryness as a side effect and is best used once nightly and applied sparingly. Mild photosensitivity may occur initially.

Figure 1-6

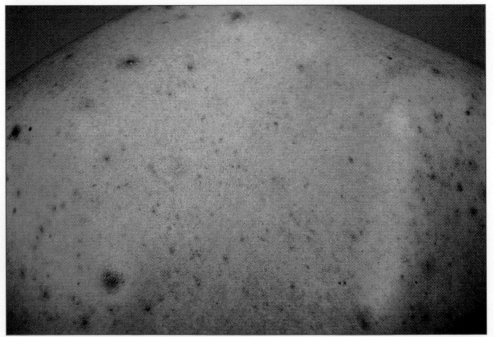

Inflammatory papulonodular acne of the back.

Figure 1-7

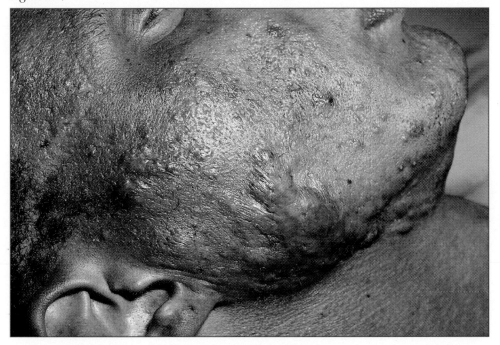

Extensive scarring from long-standing poorly controlled nodular acne.

Patients should be cautioned that this agent may initially exacerbate acne, although improvement will follow. Some patients may require 1 to 2 months of therapy to become accustomed to this agent. As with tretinoin, we encourage patients to begin with small amounts of drug and gradually increase the quantity as the skin becomes tolerant. Adapalene can be applied by patients at the same time as other topical agents and does not seem to be inactivated in this case.

TAZAROTENE   Tazarotene (Tazorac) is best considered a topical agent for psoriasis rather than a therapy of choice for acne vulgaris. Tazarotene is the only topical agent available in the United States to be labeled as Pregnancy Category X: Proven fetal risks are present that outweigh any possible benefit. Accordingly, if the clinician chooses to use this agent, pregnancy counseling and monitoring are useful. Because of this problem and the extreme expense of this agent, few patients are good candidates for tazarotene for acne.

ACIDS

AZALEIC ACID   Azaleic acid (Azalex) is a newly available agent with antibacterial and antikeratinization effects. Whether this agent is superior to other acid products is not clear, as few comparative trials have been performed in acne vulgaris. A

Figure 1-8

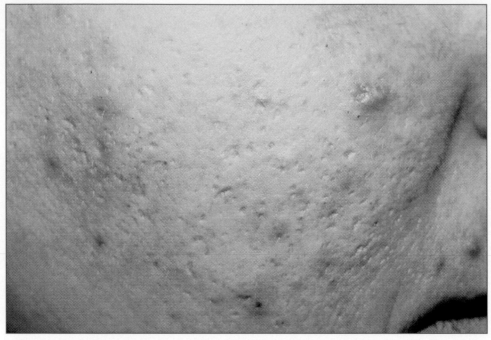

"Ice pick" scarring from papular and nodular acne.

useful side effect is that azaleic acid can cause hypopigmentation, which some patients with postinflammatory hyperpigmentation appreciate. It may play a role in reducing inflammatory papules as well. It is best applied once daily and sparingly. Azaleic acid may cause burning and stinging in people with sensitive skin.

SALICYLIC ACID   Another common agent found in over-the-counter (OTC) washes (e.g., Neutrogena Oil Free Acne Wash, SALac) is salicylic acid. This agent has comedolytic activity and, beyond drying, is generally well tolerated. Many cosmetic agents marketed for wrinkling now contain small to modest amounts of salicylic acid.

This agent may be particularly useful in patients with large numbers of comedones. Salicylic acid can cause burning, peeling, and irritation. It is best tolerated by those with normal to oily skin.

GLYCOLIC AND LACTIC ACIDS   Glycolic and lactic acids have no demonstrated activity in treating acne vulgaris but are likely to be effective. When bioavailable acid is present, hydrolysis of the skin may occur and the antiacne activity is likely to be similar to that of salicylic acid. These agents generally are applied in lotions, creams, or gels but may be applied in stronger concentrations as a peel. Many glycolic and lactic acids products sold OTC or from cosmetic counters contain no bioavailable acid.

Figure 1-9

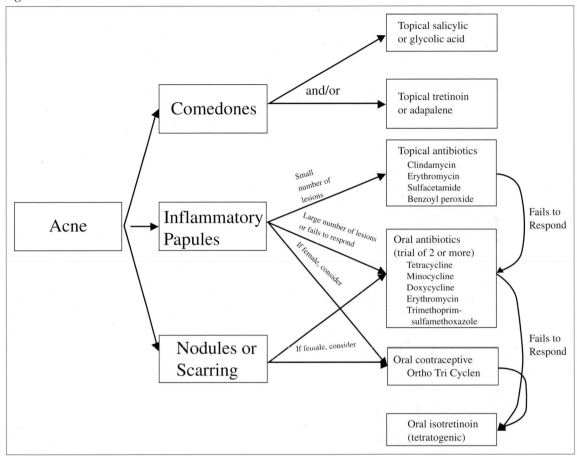

Algorithm for acne vulgaris.

ANTIBIOTIC AGENTS

BENZOYL PEROXIDE Benzoyl peroxide is a common and useful antibacterial agent that is available in both OTC forms and prescription forms. Resistance to this agent does not appear to build over time. Gels, creams, lotions, and washes generally are supplied in concentrations of 2.5 to 10%. Some products are extremely drying (e.g., Desquam-X) and are excellent for patients with excessively oily skin. By contrast, some are very well tolerated by those with dry skin (e.g., Desquam-E, Benzac AC). Benzoyl peroxide is also available mixed with erythromycin (Benzamycin); this is an agent with a limited shelf life.

It is unclear whether 10% concentrations are more effective than are 2.5% concentrations. It is clear, however, that benzoyl peroxide is a potent bleaching agent with the ability to permanently bleach clothing, bedsheets, towels, and any colored material with which it comes in contact. Washes or bars such as Benzac AC wash and Panoxyl Bar can be helpful in this regard, since the product is removed before it has the ability to bleach clothing.

ERYTHROMYCIN   Erythromycin is an inexpensive product that is available as pads, gels, solutions, and ointments. Most erythromycin products are well tolerated and efficacious. The solutions and gels tend to be somewhat drying, a benefit for acne treatment in youths but a potential problem for adults. Certain gels can clump and cause facial foundations to be applied unevenly. It is best applied once to twice daily.

CLINDAMYCIN   Clindamycin is employed frequently in preparations for acne. This antibiotic is available as pads, gels, solutions, and lotions. Because some of these products (gel and lotion) are water-based, they tend to be well tolerated by patients. It is best applied once to twice daily.

COMBINATION ANTIBIOTIC AGENTS   Multiple antibiotics may be used in combination, such as erythromycin and benzoyl peroxide (applied to the patient at the same time from two containers or as the single product Benzamycin). No commercially available combination product for clindamycin is available, but one may exist in the near future. Combination products such as Benzamycin should be considered only for patients who use topical medications rapidly. For patients who use these agents sparingly or intermittently, the benzoyl peroxide destroys the other antibiotic, rendering the agent ineffective. Another therapy, such as a topical retinoid agent, may be added to a regimen of topical antibiotics.

Systemic Therapies

ANTIBIOTIC AGENTS

TETRACYCLINE AND ERYTHROMYCIN   Tetracycline and erythromycin decrease the number of *P. acnes* on the skin's surface and have anti-inflammatory effects. They often are given in initial doses of 500 to 1000 mg/d orally (250 to 500 mg bid) and adjusted to higher or lower doses according to the response. The most common side effects of tetracycline include mild photosensitivity, staining of permanent teeth in children under 9 years of age, and *Candida* vulvovaginitis. Erythromycin causes no photosensitivity but may cause gastrointestinal upset and *Candida* vulvovaginitis. Most patients can tolerate these agents, but not all compliant patients experience clinical benefit. Although the risk is small, tetracycline should not be administered to pregnant women and young children.

MINOCYCLINE AND DOXYCYCLINE   These tetracycline derivatives are better tolerated than are tetracycline and erythromycin. They are often useful for the treatment of acne vulgaris in doses ranging from 100 to 200 mg/d orally. Minocycline (Minocin) may cause the uncommon possible side effects of blue-black pigmentation and vestibulitis. Extremely rarely, minocycline agents may produce pseudotumor cerebri. Doxycycline (Monodox) is likely to be equally effective but is a potent photosensitizer. Both agents may induce *Candida* vulvovaginitis. These agents should not be administered to pregnant women.

TRIMETHOPRIM-SULFAMETHOXAZOLE   Sulfa antibiotics such as Bactrim or Septra are often effective in the treatment of acne vulgaris but should be limited to use in cases resistant to other antibiotics because of the potential side effects of photosensitivity and allergic skin reactions. Teenagers sometimes have difficulty swallowing the large pills of the "DS" formulations. We usually employ this agent as one DS pill bid. This agent should not be administered to pregnant women. As with other systemic antibiotic agents, these agents may induce *Candida* vulvovaginitis.

HORMONAL THERAPIES

ORAL CONTRACEPTIVES   Ethinyl estradiol in combination with cyproterone acetate, desogesterol, or gestodene may improve acne in many women. The oral contraceptive Tricyclen has been approved by the U.S. Food and Drug Administration as the only hormonal acne therapy. Tricyclen helps a minority of female acne patients, particularly those with perimenstrual acne flares and/or menstrual irregularity. The side effects are similar to those seen with other oral contraceptive agents. These agents should not be administered to pregnant women.

ANTIANDROGENIC AGENTS   No antiandrogens have been approved in the United States for the treatment of acne vulgaris. In other countries, combination estrogenic and antiandrogenic hormonal therapy is employed widely. Some clinicians in the United States employ spironolactone. Clinicians should carefully read the prescribing information for this agent and discuss its use with patients.

RETINOID THERAPY

ISOTRETINOIN (ACCUTANE)   Isotretinoin is a synthetic oral retinoid that is the single most effective agent for treating acne. It is administered in doses of 0.5 to 2.0 mg/kg per day for severe acne that has been resistant to several different oral antibiotics and in patients with severe acne who are unable to tolerate standard treatments. A daily course of 1.0 mg/kg for 16 to 20 weeks often produces a remission that lasts months to years in the majority of patients. Isotretinoin is not a cure for acne. Overall, one-fourth of patients will need to repeat a course of isotretinoin in the future, one-half will need other forms of therapy (topical agents or oral antibiotics), and one-fourth will need no further therapy.

All patients who take isotretinoin experience side effects. Preparing patients for side effect management before administration produces more satisfied patients. Patients unwilling to experience common side effects such as cheilitis and xerosis should not initiate treatment. The side effects are similar to the hypervitaminosis A syndrome and limit use to more severe or scarring cases of acne. Most patients experience cheilitis, xerosis, conjunctivitis, and pruritus, and many may have bone and joint pain, headaches, epistaxis, and nausea. Uncommon complaints include alopecia, headaches, depression, and night blindness. Extremely rarely, this agent may produce pseudotumor cerebri. Laboratory monitoring is required, and the clinician should pay particular attention to pregnancy tests, the presence of hypertriglyceridemia, and elevated liver transaminase tests. Some clinicians choose to monitor a great number of laboratory tests in addition to the ones mentioned above, including urinalysis, complete blood count, and electrolytes. There are no firm guidelines suggesting the minimum or maximum number of laboratory tests required. The authors have treated patients who stated that they desired treatment with isotretinoin but refused to undergo laboratory monitoring. Without appropriate monitoring, this agent is not safe to administer, and the clinician should refuse to prescribe it.

The most important concerns in giving isotretinoin are the possible teratogenic effects on the fetus. This agent is highly teratogenic, and one capsule may be sufficient to induce severe fetal abnormalities. Sexually active women who use unreliable forms of birth control are poor candidates for this therapy. A thorough informed consent is essential before initiating therapy. Dual-method contraception control in women at risk of becoming pregnant should be started at least 1 month before beginning therapy and should continue 1 month after the cessation of therapy. The only women with 100 percent reliable contraception are those who have undergone a hysterectomy and those who engage in no sexual activity (not necessarily those who report no activity). We go through the informed consent process for women who have undergone a tubal ligation and women whose sexual partners have had vasectomies. These sterilization techniques are highly but not totally effective. In sexually active women, a negative pregnancy test should be obtained before beginning isotretinoin therapy and at monthly intervals during the treatment course.

TRETINOIN AND ACITRETIN   Other retinoid agents are available for systemic use and probably are effective, but they are not indicated or recommended for the treatment of acne vulgaris.

Intralesional Therapy

INTRALESIONAL INJECTION

Patients with a few, painful acne nodules can be helped acutely with intralesional injection of triamcinolone 3 mg/mL. Often, 0.1 to 0.3 mL injected with a 30-gauge needle is sufficient to decrease the pain and swelling in a nodule rapidly. Patients who frequently require intralesional therapy need ongoing systemic therapy or have to change the current systemic therapy to a more effective approach.

Bibliography

Brogden RN, Goa KE: Adapalene: A review of its pharmacological properties and clinical potential in the management of mild to moderate acne. *Drugs* 53:511, 1997.
DeGroot HE, Friedlander SF: Update on acne. *Curr Opin Pediatr* 10:381, 1998.

Eichenfield LF, Leyden JJ: Acne: Current concepts of pathogenesis and approach to rational treatment. *Pediatrician* 18:218, 1991.

Healy E, Simpson N: Acne vulgaris. *Br Med J,* 308:831, 1994.

Katsambas AD: Why and when the treatment of acne fails: What to do. *Dermatology* 196:158, 1998.

Koo JY, Smith LL: Psychologic aspects of acne. *Pediatr Dermatol* 8:185, 1991.

Leyden JJ: New understandings of the pathogenesis of acne. *J Am Acad Dermatol* 32:S15, 1995.

Leyden JJ: Oral isotretinoin: How can we treat difficult acne patients? *Dermatology* 195 (suppl 1):29, 1997.

Leyden JJ: The role of isotretinoin in the treatment of acne: Personal observations. *J Am Acad Dermatol* 39:S45, 1998.

Lowe JG: The stigma of acne. *Br J Hosp Med* 49:809, 1993.

Lucky AW: A review of infantile and pediatric acne. *Dermatology* 196:95, 1998.

Mackrides PS, Shaughnessy AF: Azalaic acid therapy for acne. *Am Fam Phys* 54:2457, 1996.

Meynadier J, Alirezai M: Systemic antibiotics for acne. *Dermatology* 196:135, 1998.

Nguyen QH, Kim YA, Schwartz RA: Management of acne vulgaris. *Am Fam Phys* 50:89, 99, 1994.

Shalita AR: Clinical aspects of acne. *Dermatology* 196:93, 1998.

Shaw JC: Antiandrogen and hormonal treatment of acne. *Dermatol Clin* 14:803, 1996.

Spellman MC, Pincus SH: Efficacy and safety of azalaic acid and glycolic acid combination therapy compared with tretinoin therapy for acne. *Clin Therap* 20:711, 1998.

Sykes NL Jr, Webster GF: Acne: A review of optimum treatment. *Drugs* 48:59, 1994.

Thiboutot DM: An overview of acne and its treatment. *Cutis* 57:8, 1996.

Weiss JS: Current options for the topical treatment of acne vulgaris. *Pediatr Dermatol* 14:480, 1997.

Weiss JS, Shavin JS: Adapalene for the treatment of acne vulgaris. *J Am Acad Dermatol* 39:S50, 1998.

Winston MH, Shalita AR: Acne vulgaris: Pathogenesis and treatment. *Pediatr Clin North Am* 38:889, 1991.

Atopic Dermatitis

Background

Atopic dermatitis (atopic eczema) is an idiopathic hereditary disorder in which there is increased reactivity of the skin to irritants and allergens. Patients with atopic dermatitis are likely to be affected by asthma and allergic rhinitis. Psychological, climatic, and behavioral factors may exacerbate the disease.

Epidemiology

The incidence of atopic dermatitis is unknown, but the prevalence has been reported to be as low as 2 percent and as high as 20 percent; a likely range is 5 to 10 percent. A personal or family history of atopic dermatitis, allergic rhinitis, or asthma is obtained in about one-third to half of all cases. If one parent has atopic dermatitis, the risk in a child is 20 percent; two atopic parents raise the risk to 50 percent. The age of onset is 2 to 6 months in most cases, and onset occurs in the first year of life in 60 percent. Onset before age 2 months may occur, but patients at this age are unable to scratch effectively, and so the typical signs are diminished. Although not common, the disease may start at any age later in life. Spontaneous remissions may occur in childhood, but affected patients continue to have sensitive skin.

Pathophysiology

Our understanding of the basic pathophysiologic mechanisms that cause atopic dermatitis is limited. A broad spectrum of immunologic abnormalities exist in atopic dermatitis. Atopic patients often have increased serum total IgE and specific IgE antibody to ingested or inhaled antigens. Specific T cell overproduction and activity play a vital role in the generation of inflammation in those with atopic dermatitis, and atopic patients overproduce activated T cells that migrate to the skin because of their cutaneous lymphocyte-associated antigen ligand. There are also decreased numbers and activity levels of suppressor T cells.

Xerosis, or dry skin, is a manifestation of chronic atopic dermatitis. Xerotic skin is more easily irritated than is well-hydrated skin, and decreased amounts of ceramides and other lipids seem to be associated with increased transepidermal water loss. Atopic xerosis shows various stratum corneum functional impairments, probably reflecting increased epidermal proliferation resulting from a low-level ongoing dermatitis.

Although widely recommended and accepted as dogma, milk avoidance has not been rigorously proved to decrease atopic dermatitis. Maternal allergen avoidance during pregnancy and lactation is unlikely to play a major prophylactic role. Reactivity to house dust mite allergen varies from 6 percent to 85 percent, depending on the testing method. In patients with severe disease, prophylactic measures to decrease house dust mite numbers can reduce clinical disease severity.

Clinical infection is very common in atopic dermatitis, and in some of these cases impaired neutrophil chemotaxis has been demonstrated. Atopic patients are predisposed toward developing superinfection with *Staphylococcus spp.*

Clinical Features

In childhood, favored sites include the antecubital and popliteal fossae, neck, wrists and ankles, trunk, face, periauricular area, and scalp (Figs. 2-1 through 2-5). The trunk is the most common site in both infants and children. In adolescents and adults, the distribution is similar; particularly common areas include the antecubital and popliteal fossae and hands. In early disease, erythema and fine scaling are present. With additional scratching or rubbing, papules and lichenified plaques appear, often with visible excoriation. In persons of African ancestry, a follicular papular lichenification pattern is particularly common.

Vesiculation may occur independently or may accompany superinfection with staphylococci or herpes simplex.

Figure 2-1

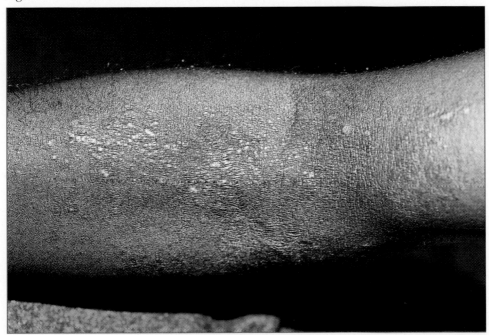

Antecubital fossa lichenification and scaling in chronic atopic dermatitis. Many darker-skinned patients have more hyperpigmentation than erythema.

Figure 2-2

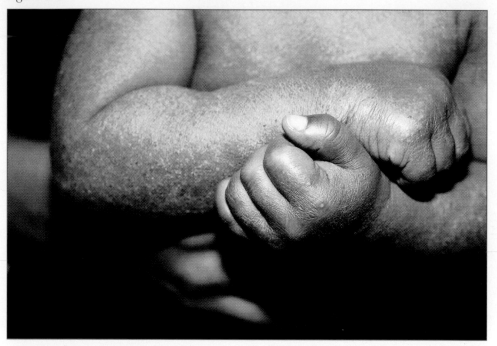

Diffuse involvement in a child caught in the act of scratching.

Atopic or Atopic-Resembling Disease as Part of Other Diseases

An eruption resembling atopic dermatitis with or without other atopic disorders and sometimes with raised IgE levels may be found in several syndromes. When the disease presents with unusual features such as failure to respond to intensive therapy and extensive perianal involvement or is accompanied by unusual systemic features, or if the features of a genetic or immunologic disorder coexist, the disease may be part of a syndrome. Recurrent unexplained infections, failure to thrive, other developmental abnormalities, and hepatosplenomegaly should be investigated. The following conditions are in this differential diagnosis:

• Acrodermatitis enteropathica
• Agammaglobulinemia
• Anhidrotic ectodermal defect
• Ataxia-telangiectasia
• Cystic fibrosis heterozygote

- Dubowitz syndrome
- Experimental histidine depletion
- Glucagonoma syndrome
- Gluten-sensitive enteropathy
- Hearing loss (genetic)
- Histidinemia
- Hyper-IgE syndrome
- Hurler syndrome
- Letterer-Siwe syndrome
- Nephrotic syndrome
- Netherton's syndrome
- Phenylketonuria
- Selective IgA deficiency
- Wiskott-Aldrich syndrome

Figure 2-3

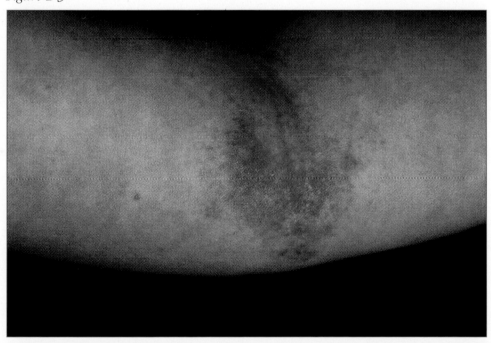

Acute flare of atopic dermatitis in the anticubital fossa.

Figure 2-4

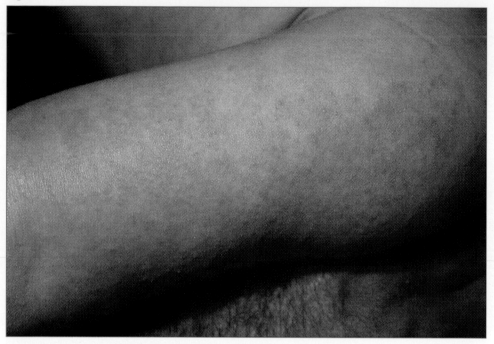

More subtle erythema indicates areas of early involvement of dermatitis.

Prognosis

Spontaneous remissions during childhood are well known, but active disease may persist through the first several decades of life. Atopic patients may be likely to get other dermatitides, such as hand dermatitis, later in life, and it may be wise for these patients to choose career paths (e.g., beauticians, dishwashers, mechanics) that avoid excessive exposure to irritants.

Treatment

In general, we recommend the treatment approach outlined in Fig. 2-6. As non-corticosteroidal topical therapies become available, this algorithm is likely to change.

Emollients and Behavioral Changes

Stopping the frequent use of harsh soaps and detergents on affected skin is an important part of the therapeutic intervention. Mild, nondrying soaps and soap substitutes (Dove, Alpha Keri, Basis, Lowila, Cetaphil, and Neutrogena) diminish the removal of epidermal lipids. The frequency of bathing should be limited as much as is reasonable. Many clinicians and patients anecdotally believe that clothing detergents exacerbate the condition, and enzyme-containing detergents are particularly bad for atopic skin. There is no evidence suggesting that these clothing detergent recommendations are helpful.

The regular use of emollients such as Moisturel improves disease severity in patients with atopic dermatitis; combined with other therapies, this is particularly efficacious. Emollients also may have a corticosteroid-sparing effect. Immediately after bathing is an important time to apply emollients to seal in the water in the hydrated epidermis. Emollients are particularly important to maintain remission. When over-the-counter (OTC) emollients alone are insufficient to maintain remission, one should consider the use of ammonium lactate 12% cream (Lac-Hydrin). Ammonium lactate can help remove xerotic skin and help restore the normal epidermal barrier function.

Figure 2-5

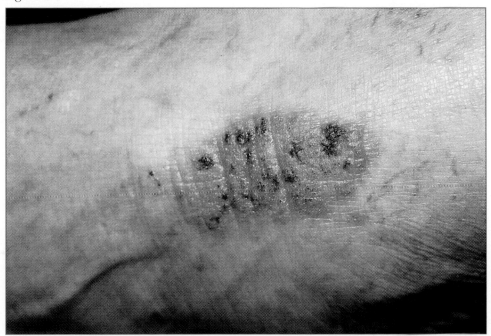

Lichenification and crusts from recent excoriation indicate the chronicity and severe pruritus of atopic dermatitis.

Figure 2-6

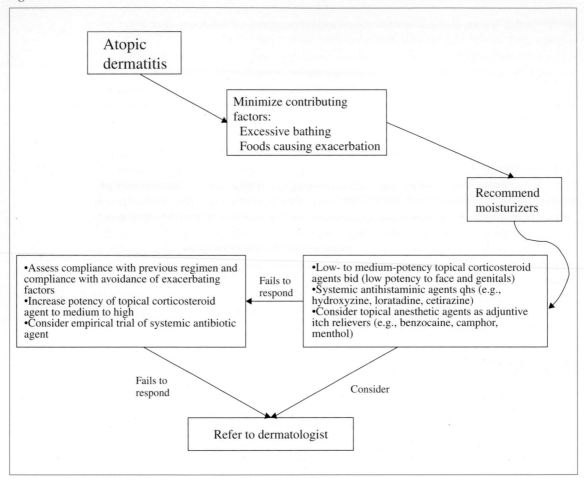

Algorithm for atopic dermatitis.

Diet

Some studies show that a minority of patients with atopic dermatitis may flare when exposed to certain foods. Parents are often aware of these individual inciting agents. Studies of long-term food avoidance show no benefit on the disease severity of atopic dermatitis. Therefore, the role of food counseling is uncertain in this disease. Strict food elimination diets have no scientific justification. If specific foods seem to make atopic dermatitis flare, those foods should be avoided. Allergy testing on patients strongly suspected of having food allergies could be considered, but atopic patients tend to overreact to many nonpathogenic stimuli.

Miscellaneous Measures

Increasing ambient humidity in dry environments may help xerosis and prevent recurrences. Heat often exacerbates the disease, and so keeping the environment cool in winter and summer should be encouraged. A scrupulously clean environment relatively free of house dust mites may help minimize exacerbations. Coarse woolen clothing may exacerbate the disease and should be avoided, but fine wool may be tolerated. Itching should be treated early. The application of antipruritic agents before erythema and lichenification develop results in an exceptionally rapid response.

Systemic Therapy

ANTIBIOTIC AGENTS

Systemic antibiotics are necessary when secondary infection is present, but some clinicians anecdotally believe that systemic antibiotic agents may be beneficial for severe exacerbations. This belief is supported by the finding of greater than normal staphylococcal counts on diseased skin in atopic patients. Therapeutically, the use of antibiotics was not borne out in a clinical trial comparing flucloxacillin with placebo. In that trial, the antibiotic did not improve the symptoms or clinical appearance of atopic dermatitis and only temporarily changed skin colonization by staphylococcus. If clinicians choose an antibiotic agent, the agent chosen should be aimed at reducing staphylococcal colonization; one should consider erythromycin (Emycin), azithromycin (Zithromax), dicloxacillin, and cephalexin (Keflex).

ANTIHISTAMINES

By virtue of their sedative action, antihistamines may help prevent nighttime scratching behavior. Bedtime doses of chlorpheniramine (Chlor-Trimeton), diphenhydramine (Benadryl), hydroxyzine (Atarax), and trimeprazine (Temaril) may be particularly helpful in diminishing the itch-scratch cycle at night. Among the less-sedating antihistamines, cetirizine (Zyrtec) and loratidine (Claritin) are likely to be the most beneficial. In addition to antihistaminic effects, cetirizine inhibits inflammatory mediator release and diminishes eosinophil and neutrophil migration. Loratidine is also likely to have some anti-inflammatory action.

SYSTEMIC CORTICOSTEROID AGENTS

Corticosteroid agents such as short-term prednisone or prednisolone (0.5 to 1 mg/kg per day) or the systemic equivalent for 1 to 2 weeks may help calm a severe exacerbation. Generally, patients with over 50 percent body surface area involvement that has not cleared despite continuous use of topical corticosteroid agents should be considered for this treatment. Many dermatologists believe that there is never a justification for using systemic corticosteroid agents. Even when it is effective, long-term use usually cannot be justified because of the inevitable and profound side effects, including osteopenia, cataracts, diabetes, and cutaneous atrophy. When systemic corticosteroid agents are used, a plan to discontinue therapy as soon as possible should be made explicit.

MISCELLANEOUS THERAPIES

Other immunologic agents, such as cyclosporine (Neoral), have demonstrated efficacy in severe and treatment-refractory atopic dermatitis. Short-term use such as 2 to 4 weeks at 5 mg/kg per day results in rapid improvement in itching and other aspects of clinical disease severity. Long-term use may be indicated in an exceptional patient who cannot be controlled with multiple other modalities. Patients who should be considered for cyclosporine are those with extensive disease, often with more than 50 percent total body surface area involvement, who have not responded to topical therapy alone. These patients probably will require ongoing treatment, and cyclosporine therapy over months to years is safer than long-term systemic corticosteroidal therapy. Although its side effects may be preferable to those of long-term corticosteroid agents, cyclosporine may cause profound immunosuppression, nephrotoxicity, hypertension, and other severe side effects.

Herbal remedies have some promoters, but given the high placebo response rate, it is likely that most activity in herbal remedies occurs through the placebo effect. However, there is good experimental evidence suggesting that some herbal remedies are highly efficacious. Traditional Chinese herbal therapy administered as a daily decoction of a formula containing 10 herbs, which was to be found beneficial in open studies, was tested for 2 months in a double-blind placebo-controlled study of adults. Despite poor palatability, itching and disease severity clearly improved and no side effects were reported.

Topical Therapy

OVERVIEW

Some patients have brief disease flares that can be controlled rapidly, and long remission times may be achieved. Other patients may need ongoing topical therapy for months to years. When long-term therapy is indicated, clinicians should continue to minimize long-term exposure to corticosteroid agents.

CORTICOSTEROID AGENTS

Corticosteroid agents are the mainstay of topical therapy. Short-term (2 to 8 weeks) administration of these agents is particularly useful in stopping the itch-scratch cycle. That is, patients itch, and so they scratch, damaging the skin, and so they itch more. Thus, the itch-scratch cycle perpetuates itself. We recommend twice-daily application of all agents. The stronger the relative potency is, the more likely it is that the agent will be effective (Table 2-1). The greater the potency, the greater the risk of local and systemic untoward effects.

There is no limit to the amount of body surface area that may be treated with topical corticosteroid agents. However, the greater the quantity, the greater the expense and the risk of adrenal-pituitary axis suppression. We prescribe mild corticosteroid agents such as hydrocortisone or medium-potency agents such as triamcinolone by the pound quantity. One pound is required for twice-daily use by an adult to apply to the total body for 1 week. Most patients require less than this, as they have less surface area involved. Moreover, occlusion with

Table 2-1

Corticosteroid Potency

Group I: Superhigh potency	Betamethasone diproprionate (Diprolene ointment, gel, solution)
	Clobetasol (Temovate cream, ointment, emollient cream, gel, solution)
	Diflorasone diacetate (Psorcon ointment)*
	Halobetasol (Ultravate cream, ointment)
Group II: Potent	Amcinonide (Cyclocort ointment)
	Betamethasone diproprionate (Diprolene AF cream)
	Desoximetasone (Topicort cream, ointment, gel)
	Diflorasone diacetate (Florone ointment or Psorcon cream)
	Fluocinonide (Lidex cream, ointment, gel, solution)
	Halcinonide (Halog cream, ointment, solution)
	Mometasone furoate (Elocon ointment)
Group III: Midpotent	Amcinonide (Cyclocort cream, lotion)
	Betamethasone diproprionate (Diprosone cream)
	Betamethasone valerate (Valisone ointment)
	Diflorasone diacetate (Florone or Maxiflor cream)
	Fluocinonide (Lidex E cream)
	Fluticasone proprionate (Cutivate ointment)
	Triamcinolone acetonide (Aristocort A ointment)
Group IV: Midpotent	Fluocinolone acetonide (Synalar ointment)
	Flurandrenolide (Cordran ointment)
	Hydrocortisone valerate (Westcort ointment)
	Mometasone furoate (Elocon cream)
	Triamcinolone acetonide (Aristocort and Kenalog cream)
Group V: Midpotent	Betamethasone diproprionate (Diprosone lotion)
	Betamethasone valerate (Valisone cream)
	Fluocinolone acetonide (Synalar cream)
	Flurandrenolide (Cordran SP cream)
	Fluticasone proprionate (Cutivate cream)
	Hydrocortisone butyrate (Locoid cream)
	Hydrocortisone valerate (Westcort cream)
	Triamcinolone acetonide (Kenalog lotion)
Group VI: Mild potency	Aclometasone diproprionate (Aclovate cream, ointment)
	Betasmethasone valerate (Valisone Lotion)
	Desonide (Desowen or Tridesilon cream, ointment, lotion)
	Fluocinolone acetonide (Synalar solution, Dermasmoothe FS oil)
Group VII: Low potency	Hydrocortisone, dexamethasone, flumethasone, prednisolone, methylprednisolone

* Less potent than group I agents.

plastic wrap or even a diaper increases the efficacy and limits the side effects of treatment.

Hydrocortisone alone may be effective in mildly affected children and adults. Failure of hydrocortisone to clear atopic dermatitis is well known, and despite its safety, topical hydrocortisone can suppress the hypothalamic-adrenal-pituitary axis. Other low-potency corticosteroid agents, including desonide (DesOwen) and aclometasone (Aclovate), are frequently more effective than hydrocortisone. Medium-potency corticosteroid agents such as hydrocortisone valerate (Westcort), triamcinolone acetonide (Kenalog), and fluticasone proprionate (Cutivate) can be beneficial in children and adults with more severe disease. Potent and superpotent corticosteroid agents are appropriate when other treatments have failed or when patients have thick, lichenified plaques. Examples of these stronger agents are halcinonide (Halog), fluocinonide (Lidex), mometasone furoate (Elocon), halobetasol (Ultravate), and clobetasol (Temovate).

Patients with chronic atopic dermatitis who use these corticosteroid agents continuously should be monitored for local side effects. A useful rule for the clinician is to use the least potent corticosteroid agent that works.

TOPICAL ANTIBIOTIC AGENTS

Topical antimicrobial agents alone play a very small role in the treatment of atopic dermatitis, but when combined with corticosteroid agents they may be effective. A trial has demonstrated that a regimen of topical mupirocin and hydrocortisone daily is as effective as hydrocortisone twice daily. It is unclear whether hydrocortisone once a day would have been as effective as mupirocin combined with hydrocortisone.

ANESTHETICS

Some patients benefit from adjunctive therapy with local anesthetic agents such as benzocaine (Lanacane) and pramoxine (Pramagel, Pramasone). These agents are likely to produce synergy with corticosteroid agents, and clinicians should consider their use to minimize corticosteroid requirements. Although these agents are potential sensitizers, it is known that they are no more allergenic than are topical corticosteroid agents.

IMMUNOMODULATING AGENTS

In the next several years, corticosteroid-sparing topical anti-inflammatory drugs such as tacrolimus and other drugs probably will become commercially available. Their greatest utility will be in patients with chronic atopic dermatitis who require long-term topical approaches and are at the greatest risk of atrophy. Topical tacrolimus (Protopic) appears to be highly effective in treating atopic dermatitis, yet it completely lacks the ability to thin the skin that is associated with all corticosteroid agents. It is applied twice daily to the affected areas. The only major problem seen with this agent has been mild and transient stinging upon application, which improves within a few days. Tacrolimus is unlikely to replace topical corticosteroid agents, but it could be used synergistically with those agents to minimize their requirement. Because of its safety compared with phototherapy and systemic therapy, tacrolimus may decrease the number of patients requiring such intervention.

Other Approaches

Some patients with recalcitrant disease may benefit from phototherapy. Ultraviolet A (UVA), ultraviolet B (UVB), combination UVA and UVB, and psoralen photochemotherapy (PUVA) have been used with beneficial results. Ultraviolet therapy cannot be used in young children but can be used in older children and adults. It generally is reserved for patients with severe and refractory disease that might otherwise require systemic treatment with cyclosporine. This treatment requires visiting phototherapeutic facilities three to five times per week for 2 to 3 months. Accordingly, patients need to be highly motivated and have generalized disease before this treatment is feasible.

Behavioral therapy and other psychological treatments of the patient or family can lead to long-term improvement in skin disease severity. These treatments should be considered adjuncts to dermatologic treatment.

Bibliography

Ainley-Walker PF, Patel L, David TJ: Side to side comparison of topical treatment in atopic dermatitis. *Arch Dis Child* 79:149, 1998.

Alaiti S, Kang S, Fiedler VC, et al: Tacrolimus (FK506) ointment for atopic dermatitis: A phase I study in adults and children. *J Am Acad Dermatol* 38:69, 1998.

Andersen PH, Bindslev-Jensen C, Mosbech H, et al: Skin symptoms in patients with atopic dermatitis using enzyme-containing detergents: A placebo-controlled study. *Acta Dermatol Venereol* 78:60, 1998.

Arkwright PD, Patel L, David TJ: Dietary management of atopic eczema: Is this justified? *Hosp Med* 59:690, 1998.

Champion RH, Parish WE: Atopic dermatitis, in Champion RH, Burton JL, Ebling FJG (eds): *Textbook of Dermatology*, 5th ed. Oxford, Blackwell, 1992, pp. 589–610.

Ewing CI, Ashcroft C, Gibbs AC, et al: Flucloxacillin in the treatment of atopic dermatitis. *Br J Dermatol* 138:1022, 1998.

Hanifin JM: Assembling the puzzle pieces in atopic inflammation. *Arch Dermatol* 132:1230, 1996.

Hanifin JM: Atopic dermatitis: New therapeutic considerations. *J Am Acad Dermatol* 24:1097, 1991.

Kim HJ, Honig PJ: Atopic dermatitis. *Curr Opin Pediatr* 10:387, 1998.

Krutmann J, Diepgen TL, Luger TA, et al: High-dose UVA1 therapy for atopic dermatitis: Results of a multicenter trial. *J Am Acad Dermatol* 38:589, 1998.

Rajka G: *Essential Aspects of Atopic Dermatitis*. Berlin, Springer-Verlag, 1989.

Reitamo S, Rissanen J, Remitz A, et al: Tacrolimus ointment does not affect collagen synthesis: Results of a single-center randomized trial. *J Invest Dermatol* 111:396, 1998.

Strange P, Skov L, Lisby S, et al: Staphylococcal enterotoxin B applied on intact normal and intact atopic skin induces dermatitis. *Arch Dermatol* 132:27, 1996.

Thestrup-Pederson K: The incidence and pathophysiology of atopic dermatitis. *J Eur Acad Dermatol Venereol* 7 (suppl 1):S3, 1996.

Wolkerstorfer A, Strobos MA, Glazenburg EJ, et al: Fluticasone propionate 0.05% cream once daily versus clobetasone butyrate 0.05% cream twice daily in children with atopic dermatitis. *J Am Acad Dermatol* 39:226, 1998.

Wulf HC, Bech-Thomsen N: A UVB phototherapy protocol with very low dose increments as a treatment of atopic dermatitis. *Photodermatol Photoimmunol Photomed* 14:1, 1998.

Psoriasis

Background

Psoriasis is an inflammatory disorder of the skin that is characterized by a variety of morphologic lesions. The most common form of psoriasis—psoriasis vulgaris—is typified by a chronic, relapsing nature and erythematous plaques covered with thick scales. Other variants, such as a pustular form, a guttate form, a diffuse erythrodermic form, and an intertriginous variant, exist. The unifying characteristics of these diverse-appearing variants include a red, scaly morphology; a histopathology characterized by epidermal hyperplasia and inflammation; and a tendency for patients to exhibit different variants at one time or at different times. This chapter focuses primarily on the most common form, psoriasis vulgaris.

Risk Factors

Psoriasis can present at any time from the first few weeks of life until 80 or more years of age. Onset is rare in infancy and uncommon in childhood; most patients experience onset in the third decade. There is a definite familial tendency to inherit psoriasis. When one parent is affected, there is a one in four chance of psoriasis in each child; with two affected parents, the rate is one in two. Most people with psoriasis, however, lack a family history of the disease. Some genetic linkage between psoriasis and the HLA-Cw6 phenotype has been demonstrated. An interrelationship also exists between psoriatic arthritis and seronegative spondyloarthropathies such as ankylosing spondylitis, Reiter's syndrome, and enteropathic arthropathies.

Pathophysiology

Psoriasis involves hyperproliferation of the epidermis in combination with the activation of inflammatory pathways. The hyperplasia of the epidermis results from both a shortened epidermal cell cycle and an increase in the proliferative cell population. The epidermal cells have additional cohesiveness, which leads to the formation of the thick scale of psoriatic plaques. The dermis probably plays a critical role in the generation of psoriasis. T-cell lymphocytes are present in large numbers in psoriatic lesions, and most of them are CD4+. Clinical improvement in response to T-cell inhibitors such as cyclosporine supports the presence of a primary immune mechanism in psoriasis. In guttate psoriasis, T-cell activation by streptococcal superantigens is thought to be involved in the pathogenesis. The underlying genetics of immune activation in psoriasis is an active area of research. Current treatments for psoriasis target both the epidermal hyperproliferation and the underlying immune pathways.

Symptoms and Physical Examination

The different varieties of psoriasis may present with an overlap of several types of lesions, and each one has a distinctive timing. Typical psoriasis is a chronic, relapsing disorder with red, thick scaly plaques in a symmetric distribution (Figs. 3-1 and 3-2). Common areas of involvement include the scalp, elbows, nails, gluteal

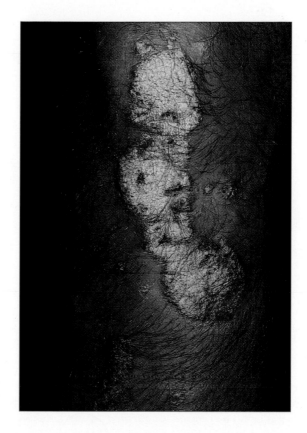

Figure 3-1

Psoriatic plaques of the knee. This well-
defined plaque has the characteristic silvery scale of psoriasis.

cleft, umbilicus, and knees (Figs. 3-3 through 3-6). Inverse psoriasis can be considered a form of psoriasis vulgaris that involves intertriginous areas; it is characterized by macerated erythematous plaques involving the intertriginous areas of the
groin, axillae, submammary area, and gluteal folds. Scaling is subtle or absent in
these lesions. Psoriatic balanitis is a form of inverse psoriasis that is represented
by erythematous plaques on the glans penis (Fig. 3-7).

Plaques may become confluent over large surface areas and range in thickness
from barely perceptible to markedly elevated. The Auspitz sign is demonstrated by
tiny areas of pinpoint bleeding when the scale is lifted from a lesion. When psoriasiform lesions are seen in other areas, the "typical" areas should be examined.
Identification in these areas confirms the diagnosis. Nail involvement is particularly
helpful in this regard; it is manifested most commonly as distal onycholysis (separation of the nail plate from the nail bed), pitting, and yellow discoloration under the nail (oil-drop lesions) (see Fig. 3-6). One nail to all nails may be involved,
and there usually are associated cutaneous lesions.

Scalp involvement also may help confirm the diagnosis of psoriasis (see Fig.
3-4). When scalp involvement is mild, it may be impossible to distinguish scalp
psoriasis from seborrheic dermatitis. The presence of psoriasis elsewhere does

Figure 3-2

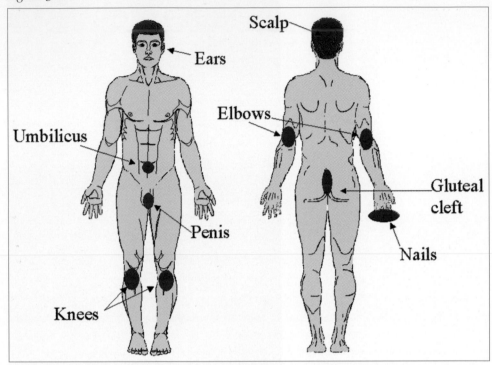

Characteristic affected areas in psoriasis. Typically, psoriasis exhibits bilateral symmetry. Common areas of involvement include the scalp, elbows, knees, nails, umbilicus, and gluteal cleft.

confirm the diagnosis of scalp psoriasis. Differentiating mild scalp psoriasis from seborrheic dermatitis is not critical. as the treatment options are identical.

Other symptoms commonly associated with psoriasis include pruritus and pain. The lesions may bleed, may appear at sites of trauma (Koebner's phenomenon), or may be very inflamed (Fig. 3-8).

Guttate psoriasis presents with the rapid onset of small, droplike psoriasiform (red and scaly) lesions that may follow an upper respiratory infection, often infection with *Streptococcus pyogenes* (Fig. 3-9). Lesions are found on the trunk and proximal extremities and often are covered with a light scale. This variant may be difficult to distinguish from pityriasis rosea. A history of preexisting psoriasis of the elbows and knees and the absence of a well-developed "Christmas tree" pattern favor psoriasis.

Erythrodermic and generalized pustular psoriasis (Fig. 3-8 through 3-10) also may arise after an infection or after the administration of medications such as beta blockers, systemic corticosteroids, and lithium in patients who previously had mild psoriasis. Marked symptoms of pruritus and arthralgias may be associated with chills, fever, and fluid and electrolyte imbalances in patients with erythrodermic psoriasis. The systemic symptoms that accompany this form of psoriasis may be severe and include fever, diarrhea, arthralgias, and leukocytosis. Because of the severity of the inflammation in generalized pustular psoriasis, patients with this condition are at risk for developing serious medical complications such as electrolyte abnormalities and fluid imbalances. Patients with erythrodermic psoriasis may have the same problems in addition to being at risk for high-output cardiac failure. A localized form of pustular psoriasis affects the palms and soles (Fig. 3-11 through 3-13). It is often a chronic, unremitting problem that can be disabling.

Psoriasis affects every dimension of health-related quality of life and can be as severe as medical disorders such as heart failure, diabetes, and depression. Psychiatric symptoms are common, and about one-third of these patients have psychiatric disease as measured by quantitative, validated instruments. These patients commonly complain about pruritus, the appearance of lesions, pain, the reactions of others, and the doctor's attitude toward psoriasis.

Beyond the significant psychologic effects, localized forms of psoriasis can be associated with joint complaints. Between one-third and one-half of patients with psoriasis have joint complaints, but only a small minority have frank psoriatic arthritis. The arthralgias and arthritis may be pauciarticular and resemble osteoarthritis in their distribution. However, the arthritis can be aggressive and joint-destroying, involving small joints in the hands and feet and rapidly leading to permanent

Figure 3-3

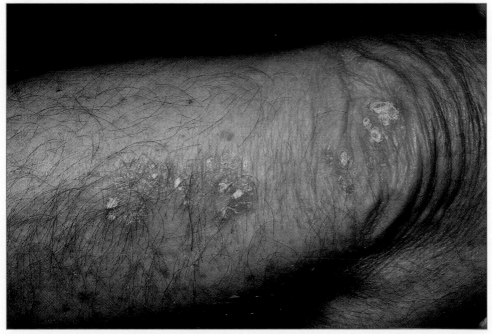

Mild psoriasis. The psoriatic plaques are red and scaly with little thickness. Topical corticosteroids, along with moisturizers and/or keratolytics, may constitute sufficient treatment for these lesions.

Figure 3-4

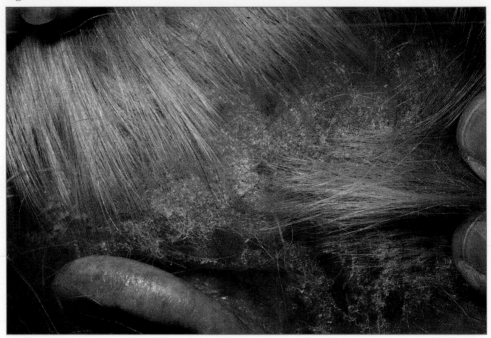

Scalp psoriasis. Scalp involvement may be difficult to see unless the clinician pulls the hair aside. Scalp psoriasis may be mild, with slight redness and scaling, or severe, with marked inflammation, as is shown here.

disability. Patients with the form of arthritis termed psoriatic arthritis mutilans have deforming abnormalities of the phalangeal joints that may result in osteolysis of the digit. Psoriatic arthritis most commonly presents as an asymmetric oligoarthropathy.

Laboratory Evaluation

The diagnosis of psoriasis usually is made on clinical grounds, and laboratory tests rarely are required. In rare instances a skin biopsy may help distinguish psoriasis from other dermatoses when there are red, scaly psoriasiform lesions in an unusual pattern and/or distribution without confirmatory nail, scalp, or other typical involvement. In these cases, punch biopsy permits the pathologist to assess the pattern of inflammation in both the superficial and the deep dermis. Special stains for fungal organisms often are performed, as the histology of psoriasis and that of superficial fungal infections (tinea) can be identical.

Figure 3-5

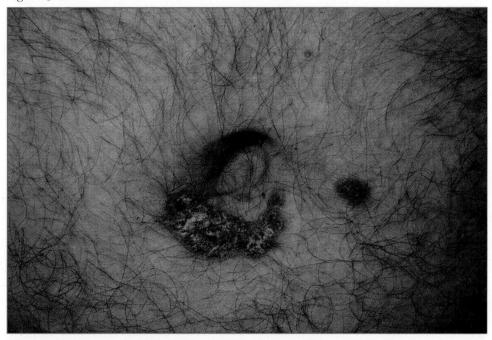

The umbilicus is a frequently affected area. This is a helpful finding when the diagnosis is uncertain.

Patients with severe pustular flares of psoriasis may present with a markedly elevated neutrophil count. The presence of fever with an extremely high white blood cell count may confuse clinicians who do not realize that psoriasis alone, in the absence of infection, can produce leukocytosis.

Treatment

Overview

Treatments for psoriasis vary widely and are dependent on the duration and extent of involvement, the psychological impact and life-style of the patient, and the cost of therapy. The treatment regimen may begin with topical therapy and advance to phototherapy or systemic therapy, according to the response and expectations of the patient. With limited disease, initial treatment with a topical corticosteroid agent combined with calcipotriene for 1 to 4 months helps clear most patients, and the corticosteroid is discontinued as quickly as possible. Phototherapy and systemic therapy generally are reserved for patients with extensive disease and patients who fail to respond to topical therapy. For any patient with destructive joint disease, systemic agents such as methotrexate and cyclosporine should be considered first-line therapy.

Topical Therapy

MOISTURIZERS AND KERATOLYTICS

Daily lubrication is a simple and important aspect of treating psoriasis. Ointments, lotions, and creams are widely available and beneficial. For patients with large amounts of scale, keratolytic preparations containing either extemporaneously compounded 2 to 6% salicylic acid in petrolatum or 12% ammonium lactate cream (Lac-Hydrin) may aid in clearing scale. The addition of keratolytics has additional utility in combination with other pharmacologic agents because the drugs can penetrate more easily through the epidermis. While keratolytics may be extremely helpful, clinicians should exercise caution in their use. Acids may irritate the skin, and salicylic acid repetitively applied to large amounts of body surface area can lead to toxic systemic levels of salicylates. Acid products should also not be used at the

Figure 3-6

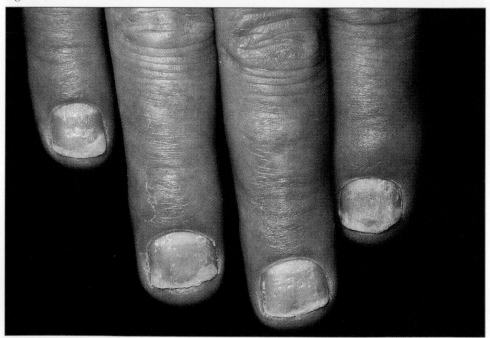

Nail changes in psoriasis. The nail changes includes small pits of the surface and separation of the nail from the nail bed. Identification of these changes is helpful when the diagnosis of psoriasis is otherwise uncertain. Fungal nail changes also must be considered. Onychomycosis is much more common on the toenails and does not cause the surface pitting seen in psoriasis.

Figure 3-7

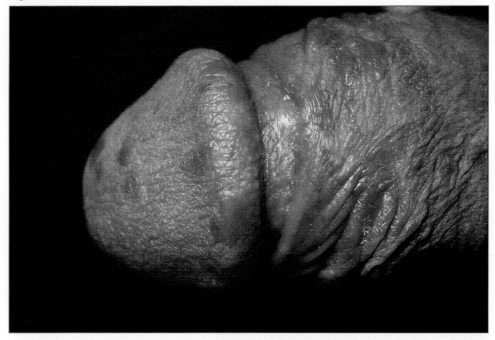

Psoriatic balanitis. Psoriasis is not uncommon on the penis. Trauma may be an exacerbating factor. Only low-potency topical corticosteroids such as 1% hydrocortisone ointment should be used in this area.

same time as topical calcipotriene, as this vitamin D analog is degraded in acid environments.

TARS

Coal tar compounds have been used for over a century to treat psoriasis. Tar is not a well-defined chemical compound and may contain as many as 10,000 separate chemicals. Although these compounds can be mildly efficacious, their efficacy is limited by local irritation and poor compliance. Tars have the advantage of being corticosteroid-sparing. However, tar preparations are malodorous and messy; that is, they stink and stain. Tar products are available as ointments, gels, creams, and shampoos. To maximize compliance and prevent the permanent staining of patients' clothes, tars usually are applied nightly. Psoriasis vulgaris responds best to tar therapy. By contrast, highly inflammatory psoriasis variants such as pustular psoriasis usually are exacerbated by tar compounds. Tar often is used in combination with ultraviolet B (UVB) light but also may be used in combination with essentially any other topical agent.

Tars may cause folliculitis and irritation in some patients, and many patients cannot tolerate any form of tar. Some components of tar are clearly oncogenic and may be absorbed systemically. It is doubtful that these compounds are clinically relevant carcinogens, but like other therapeutic agents, tars cannot be considered absolutely safe.

ANTHRALIN

Anthralin is an anti-inflammatory agent that has the advantage of being corticosteroid-sparing. As with tar, topical anthralin is a treatment in which efficacy is limited by extreme local irritation and poor compliance. Patients can develop severe contact dermatitis if anthralin products are left on the skin for prolonged periods. To minimize irritation, anthralin preparations often are applied only to the lesions (not to perilesional skin) for 10 to 30 minutes, and then the preparation is washed off. Patients must be counseled that the psoriatic plaques and the surrounding skin will turn brown, and that this coloration may persist for several weeks to a month after the discontinuation of therapy. Anthralin is available in a scalp solution as well as in cream and ointment forms.

CORTICOSTEROIDS

Topical corticosteroids frequently are used to treat psoriasis and have a number of advantages. Unlike tars and anthralin, they never cause staining and rarely cause irritation. However, psoriasis is a chronic disease that is readily treatable but never

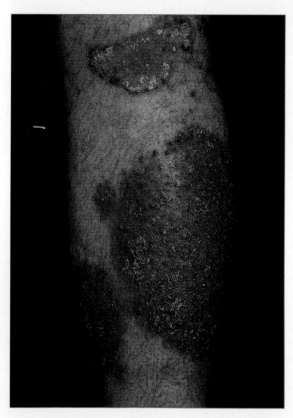

Figure 3-8

Inflamed psoriasis. Psoriasis can be quite inflamed and painful. These areas of psoriasis exhibit little scale. Irritating topical therapies and phototherapy should be avoided until the inflammation has "cooled down" from the use of a topical corticosteroid (such as 0.1% triamcinolone) ointment.

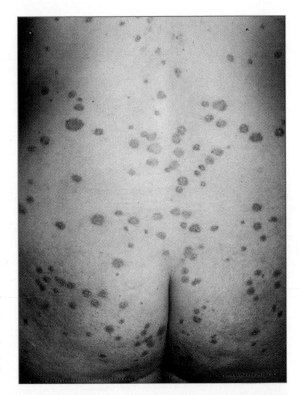

Figure 3-9

Guttate psoriasis is characterized by small, drop-shaped psoriasiform plaques. Because this is an acute variant, there is no time for the development of thick scales, and so the lesions appear redder and less thick and scaly.

curable. Accordingly, patients who use topical corticosteroid agents over months to years run a real risk of permanent atrophy, telangiectasia, and fragility of the treated skin. Also, topical corticosteroid agents decrease the remission time of phototherapy (discussed below) and predispose patients to tachyphylaxis. These agents are best used to decrease inflammation while patients are making the transition from acute treatment to long-term treatment with noncorticosteroidal approaches. Clinical synergy has been demonstrated when corticosteroids are used in combination with calcipotriene and tazarotene.

A broad range of potency levels are available for topical corticosteroids. Thick plaques on the trunk and extremities require potent agents such as fluocinonide 0.05%, clobetasol proprionate 0.05%, and betamethasone diproprionate 0.05% in an optimized vehicle, whereas treatment of the face, anogenital area, and other intertrigenous areas requires more mild agents such as 1% hydrocortisone. Extensive use of topical corticosteroids, especially high-potency corticosteroids, can place a patient at risk for hypothalamic-pituitary-adrenal axis suppression. If plaques are thick and the involvement of psoriasis is not extensive, ultrapotent topical corticosteroids (halobetasol, clobetasol, and betamethasone diproporionate in an optimized vehicle) may be used, but this generally should be limited to 4 to 8 weeks. The prescribing information for these agents limits recommended treatment to 2 to 4 weeks, but thick psoriatic plaques do not resolve in 2 weeks. When using potent topical corticosteroid agents, clinicians should try to use the smallest amount

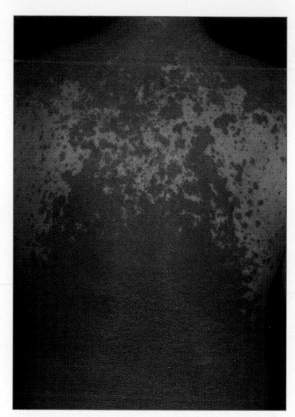

Figure 3-10

Erythrodermic psoriasis is characterized by a red eruption of all or nearly all the skin surface. There is usually little scale and few well-developed plaques. Often differentiation from other causes of erythroderma (such as drug eruptions and dermatitis) is done on the basis of a history of typical psoriatic plaques.

that results in a good response. Potent topical corticosteroids generally should not be used on the face or in intertriginous areas. Adrenal suppression has been demonstrated with as little as 2 g/d of ultrapotent agents. Occlusion increases both the effectiveness of these drugs and their potential for local and systemic side effects.

For milder cases of plaque psoriasis and for widespread disease, a midpotency compound (triamcinolone, hydrocortisone valerate, fluticasone, and similar compounds) may work well. Facial or intertriginous psoriasis may respond well to weak corticosteroid agents, including hydrocortisone, aclometasone, and desonide.

Topical corticosteroids are available in cream, ointment, lotion, and solution forms. Ointments are an excellent choice for cutaneous plaques because of their occlusive and hydrating properties, but patients may dislike the greasy consistency. Creams are more elegant, and patients may be more compliant with their use; however, they may not be ideal products for this disease. Solutions are most useful in scalp areas.

CALCIPOTRIENE

Calcipotriene is a vitamin D derivative that is available in creams, ointments, and scalp solutions. It may have effects on both keratinocyte proliferation and immune modulation in psoriasis patients. As the leading prescription agent for psoriasis treatment in the United States, it has the advantage of being cortico-steroid-sparing, and it lacks many of the irritation, odors, and staining characteristics of tar and anthralin preparation. Calcipotriene usually is used twice daily in combination with topical corticosteroids and is best for treating limited plaque psoriasis. Four weeks of this combination is normally sufficient to determine whether there will be a good clinical response. When patients approach clearing, discontinuation of the corticosteroid agent is suggested, with continuation of the calcipotriene.

Synergy has been demonstrated when topical calcipotriene is combined with UVB, psoralen with ultraviolet A photochemotherapy (PUVA), corticosteroid agents, and cyclosporine. The most common side effect is mild irritancy. In addition to better efficacy, an advantage of combining corticosteroids with calcipotriene is that combination treatment decreases the limited irritancy of calcipotriene.

Calcipotriene is available as a cream, ointment, and solution. The ointment is more effective than the cream for treating psoriatic plaques, but the cream is more elegant. The solution is useful for scalp disease. Although this is perhaps the safest single agent for the treatment of psoriasis, studies have shown alterations in calcium metabolism (hypercalcemia, hypercalciuria) with the use of more than 120 mg per week of calcipotriene and in patients with extensive disease or renal

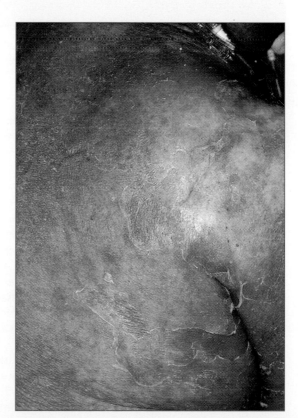

Figure 3-11

Generalized pustular psoriasis. This variant of psoriasis may present with striking inflammation, pustules, and tenderness and may be associated with systemic symptoms. The eruption may involve nearly the entire skin (erythroderma), as is shown here.

Figure 3-12

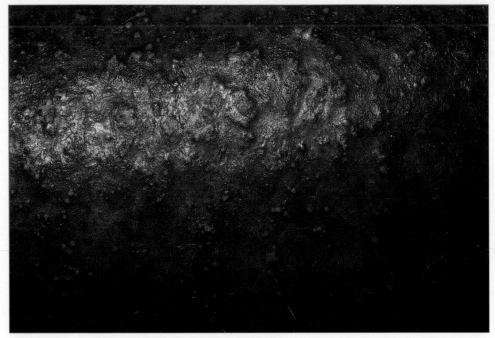

Generalized pustular psoriasis. Histologically, all forms of psoriasis have neutrophils in the superficial scale. When the collections of neutrophils are large enough, visible pustules are present, as is shown here. The pustular forms tend to be painful and are associated with systemic symptoms when severe.

impairment. Accordingly, the quantity prescribed should be limited to less than 100 g per week.

TAZAROTENE

A topical vitamin A derivative, tazarotene, is available as a topical gel for the treatment of psoriasis. Like calcipotriene, it has the advantage of being corticosteroid-sparing, and it lacks the odors and staining characteristics of tar and anthralin. It has the disadvantage of being more irritating than calipotriene, and a controlled trial comparing the two agents showed that calcipotriene is more effective than tazarotene.

Tazarotene is nevertheless a useful corticosteroid-sparing agent in treating psoriatic plaques. Tazarotene probably should be used in conjunction with a topical corticosteroid. Corticosteroid agents show a synergistic effect with tazarotene and decrease the irritancy of this agent. It is only available as a gel, but other delivery forms may be forthcoming.

The main side effect of topical tazarotene is irritancy. This agent usually is used once daily in combination with topical corticosteroids and is best for treating limited plaque psoriasis. When patients approach clearing, discontinuation of the corticosteroid agent is suggested, with continuation of the tazarotene.

Figure 3-13

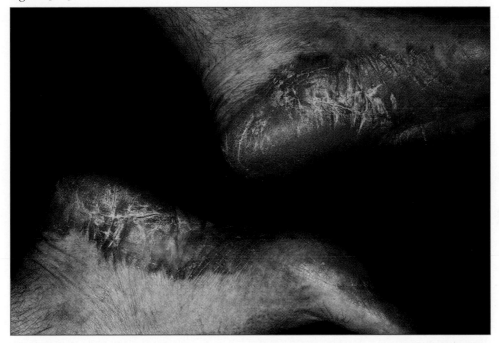

Palmoplantar pustulosis (psoriasis of the palms and soles). Because of the location on the soles and the painful character of the eruption, this form of psoriasis can be debilitating. The thickness of the skin in this area makes it difficult for topical therapy to be effective, and systemic therapy may be required.

Tazarotene is the only topical agent in the United States to be given the pregnancy Category X designation (use is contraindicated during pregnancy) by the U.S. Food and Drug Administration. Accordingly, caution should be exercised in treating women of childbearing age.

The many topical therapies for psoriasis give clinicians numerous options for initiating and continuing therapy. There are no well-established guidelines, however. Table 3-1 provides suggested approaches for treating psoriasis plaques in different situations. Special areas of psoriasis require other approaches (Table 3-2).

Phototherapy and Photochemotherapy

HELIOTHERAPY

Solar exposure has efficacy for patients who can sunbathe in the summer between 10 a.m. and 2 p.m. Unaffected areas, including the face, should be protected by hats and/or a sunscreen. Like other forms of phototherapy, this approach increases the long-term risk of cutaneous cancer and the short-term risk of burning.

Commercial tanning beds may have some efficacy in treating psoriasis. This is particularly true of tanning beds that produce large quantities of UVB. In tanning beds, the eyes must be protected during phototherapy to minimize the risk of

Table 3-1

Recommended Treatment Options for Localized Psoriasis

	INITIAL THERAPY	MAINTENANCE THERAPY
Very mild localized disease of elbows	High-potency topical corticosteroid (fluocinonide 0.05% ointment)	Moisturizers; restart topical corticosteroid with flares
Moderate localized psoriasis	Combination of super-high-potency topical corticosteroid (halobetasol 0.05%) ointment bid plus topical calcipotriene ointment bid	Once control is achieved, reduce corticosteroids to weekend use; continue calcipotriene for additional 6 weeks before tapering; reinstitute calcipotriene at earliest sign of flare
Resistant psoriasis lesions	Clobetasol proprionate ointment plus tazarotene 0.1% gel	Taper corticosteroid first to prevent rebound flare

keratitis and conjunctivitis. Heliotherapy and tanning bed therapy have not been clinically compared with more controlled phototherapeutic interventions, and so their relative efficacy is unknown.

ULTRAVIOLET B PHOTOTHERAPY

Psoriasis that is more extensive or resistant to topical preparations may respond well to UVB phototherapy (290 to 320 nm). UVB is highly effective and frequently clears patients over the course of 20 to 40 treatments. Treatment regimens usually begin at three or four times a week and may be discontinued or gradually decreased to less frequent maintenance therapy as the patient improves. Initial treatments are based on the patient's minimal erythema dose, which is a measurement of the dose of ultraviolet radiation that produces a barely perceptible erythema on the skin. Phototherapy is carried out in specialized light units. The patient often experiences redness and pain locally. There may be an increased risk of developing photoaging effects and nonmelanoma skin cancer over time. The eyes must be protected during phototherapy to minimize the risk of keratitis and conjunctivitis.

PSORALEN WITH ULTRAVIOLET A PHOTOCHEMOTHERAPY

Psoralens are natural photosensitizers that are found in some plant species. The combination of psoralens and ultraviolet A (UVA) light (320 to 400 nm) is much more effective than UVB in the treatment of psoriasis, but carries a greater risk of severe burning and carcinogenesis. The patient receives a dose of psoralen either orally or to localized areas topically; this is followed by a carefully timed exposure to UVA light. Treatments usually are done three times a week, and most patients require at least 8 to 10 treatments before improvement is noted. Psoriasis that is resistant to UVB phototherapy may respond to PUVA. The most common

Table 3-2

Psoriasis in Special Areas

Scalp	Tar shampoo daily followed by fluocinonide 0.05% solution; if not effective, topical calcipotriene solution in combination with halcinonide solution twice a day; topical tazarotene 0.01% also may be effective
Nails	No effective treatments; for onycholysis, fluocinonide or clobetasol proprionate (0.05%) solution can be allowed to wick into the space between the nail and the nail bed
Genitals	High-potency topical corticosteroids should not be used on the genitalia; 1% hydrocortisone ointment with or without topical calcipotriene ointment may be used
Ear canal	Topical corticosteroid solutions (1% hydrocortisone or fluocinolone solutions) may be used

side effect of psoralen is nausea. Careful attention must be given to protecting the patient's eyes and skin from excess ultraviolet exposure before and after treatments.

There is a high risk of nonmelanoma skin cancer after PUVA, far greater than that associated with UVB phototherapy. A recent preliminary study suggested that there may be an increased risk of melanoma with PUVA as well. These risks are sufficiently high that patients should be counseled to check on and report new or changing lesions and to have continued monitoring (complete skin examinations) annually.

In theory, PUVA treatments could be performed using oral psoralens in conjunction with tanning beds, which produce large quantities of UVA radiation. The authors strongly suggest that clinicians refrain from using this therapeutic maneuver. Death may result from excessive amounts of UVA irradiation, and adequate dosimetry is not available in community tanning salons. Similarly, we do not recommend that solar exposure be used in conjunction with oral psoralens, since solar irradiation is highly variable on a day-to-day basis.

OTHER PHOTOTHERAPEUTIC APPROACHES

Goeckerman therapy combines UVB with the application of tar-containing compounds. Ingram therapy combines UVB with anthralin. Re-PUVA is a combination of oral retinoids (acitretin or isotretinoin) with PUVA, and Re-UVB is a combination of oral retinoids with UVB. These therapies usually are available only in specialized psoriasis treatment centers.

Systemic Therapy

METHOTREXATE

Methotrexate (MTX) is a folate antagonist that is given in low weekly doses to treat psoriasis. It usually is given orally at doses ranging from 2.5 to 25 mg a week.

Initially a test dose of 5 to 10 mg is given, and if the patient tolerates the drug, doses are increased in 2.5- to 5-mg increments until results are seen.

The side effects of MTX limit its use to patients who have failed topical treatment or phototherapy. It is particularly valuable in patients with disabling cutaneous involvement or arthritis and those with pustular or erythrodermic forms of psoriasis. A thorough history and physical examination should be completed before the administration of MTX. Initial laboratory tests, including an electrolyte panel, liver function tests, and a complete blood count and differential, should be obtained before beginning therapy and at weeks 2, 4, and 8 and every 8 to 12 weeks during therapy. A urinalysis should be checked before the initiation of therapy. Common side effects of MTX include fatigue and nausea. These side effects may be minimized with the use of split dosing and the administration of daily folic acid. Uncommon side effects include oral ulcers, leukopenia, anemia, and thrombocytopenia.

MTX is uncommonly used in patients with coexisting liver disease and in those who drink alcohol heavily. Patients should avoid aspirin, nonsteroidal antiinflammatory agents, sulfa antibiotics, and alcohol while taking MTX.

Liver toxicity is a concern with MTX, and liver biopsies are recommended after a cumulative dose of 1.5 g and then with every additional 1.5 g to rule out fibrosis and cirrhosis of the liver. The liver biopsy procedure carries a real risk of serious intraabdominal hemmorhage, and so this procedure is not a trivial one. We discuss the role of liver biopsy in monitoring methotrexate toxicity with all patients before the first dose. Methotrexate should be used only by clinicians who are familiar with this agent and its side effects and are capable of monitoring for toxicity.

RETINOIDS

Oral retinoids are synthetic derivatives of vitamin A that occasionally are used to treat psoriasis that is resistant to topical therapy or in combination with UVB or PUVA. They also are used in the treatment of pustular psoriasis. Acitretin (Soriatane) has the most antipsoriatic activity but carries a pregnancy Category X designation (use is contraindicated during pregnancy) from the U.S. Food and Drug Administration. Because of its long half-life and the tremendous teratogenic potential of retinoids, acitretin has a required minimum of 3 years between the last dose and the time when pregnancy can occur. This interval should be extended indefinitely if women patients consume any alcohol during treatment because of the potential for conversion of acitretin to etretinate (a drug with an even longer half-life). Alcohol is ubiquitous and may be found in over-the-counter cough and cold remedies, and in many foods; it also may be consumed surptitiously by patients. Accordingly, it is unclear whether patients should ever become pregnant after taking acitretin.

Isotretinoin (Accutane) is not as effective as acitretin in treating psoriasis and carries a pregnancy Category X designation. Its only advantage in treating psoriasis is that it is safe to use in women of childbearing age as long as contraception is maintained 1 month before, during, and after therapy. Although it is a potent teratogen, it does not have the lingering blood and tissue levels typical of acitretin.

An informed consent process should be used for all women of childbearing age who require systemic retinoid agents.

The typical dose of acitretin is 0.5 to 1.0 mg/kg per day, and this agent can be given for 6 to 12 weeks before maximum improvement is noted. Dosing of isotretinoin is usually at 1.0 mg/kg per day. Side effects include hair loss, dry skin and lips, hypertriglyceridemia, and hepatotoxicity. As the duration of treatment increases, the frequency of side effects increases. Baseline laboratory tests should include liver function tests, triglycerides, and, in women, a pregnancy test. These tests should be repeated at appropriate intervals during therapy. A long-term side effect of retinoid therapy is the formation of extraosseous calcification of the tendons and ligaments or diffuse idiopathic skeletal hyperostosis; for this reason, radiographs of the spine and ankles should be considered yearly in patients on chronic retinoid therapy.

CYCLOSPORINE

Cyclosporine is a powerful immunosuppressant that is used only for cases of severe, treatment-resistant psoriasis. It has extraordinary efficacy and a rapid onset of action and generally is well tolerated. The usual initial doses in patients with psoriasis are 4 to 5 mg/kg per day. The advantages of cyclosporine include its lack of a teratogenic effect. Accordingly, it may be much safer to use than MTX or systemic retinoid agents in certain populations of women.

The side effects include immunosuppression, nephrotoxicity, hepatotoxicity, hypertension, and neurologic abnormalities. Patients should be monitored regularly for edema, hypertension, renal insuffienciency, and immunosuppression. This agent may be best for the acute suppression of severe disease, with a transition after several months of treatment to other agents.

Clinicians should consider whether patients who have received numerous PUVA or UVB treatments should be eligible for treatment with this agent, since it may promote cutaneous oncogenesis.

OTHER MEDICATIONS

Other secondary agents occasionally are employed in the treatment of psoriasis. Hydroxyurea is primarily a cancer chemotherapy agent that is used to treat severe, treatment-resistant psoriasis. Careful hematologic monitoring must be employed. Sulfasalazine has modest efficacy in the treatment of psoriasis and is a relatively safe agent for use in this disease.

Bibliography

Abel EA: Phototherapy. *Dermatol Clin* 13:841, 1995.

Feldman SR, Clark AR: Psoriasis, in Theirs B (ed): Office dermatology, part 1. *Med Clin North Am* 82:1135, 1982.

Fleischer AB Jr, Feldman SR, Clark AR, Reboussin DM: An uncontrolled trial of commercial tanning bed treatments for psoriasis. *J Invest Dermatol* 109:170, 1997.

Gonzalez E: PUVA for psoriasis. *Dermatol Clin* 13:851, 1995.

Guzzo D: Recent advances in the treatment of psoriasis. *Dermatol Clin* 15:59, 1997.

Jeffes EW, Weinstein GD: Methotrexate and other chemotherapeutic agents used to treat psoriasis. *Dermatol Clin* 13:875, 1995.

Kirsner RS, Federman D: Treatment of psoriasis: Role of calcipotriene. *Am Fam Phys* 52:237, 243, 1995.

Leung DY, Travers JB, Giorno R, Feldman SR: Psoriasis treatment, in Callen JP, Jorizzo JL (eds): *Current Problems in Dermatology*, vol. 10. 1998, pp. 1–40.

Norris DA, Skinner R, Aelion J, et al: Evidence for a streptococcal superantigen-driven process in acute guttate psoriasis. *J Clin Invest* 96:2106, 1995.

Ortonne JP: Aetiology and pathogenesis of psoriasis. *Br J Dermatol* 135 (suppl 49):1, 1996.

Rapp SR, Exum ML, Reboussin DM, et al: The physical, psychological and social impact of psoriasis. *J Health Psychol* 2:525, 1997.

Wieder JM, Lowe NJ: Systemic retinoids for psoriasis. *Dermatol Clin* 13:891, 1995.

Rosacea

Background

Acne rosacea is a chronic, intermittent facial eruption that is characterized in the early stages by flushing and blushing as well as by papules and papulopustules on an erythematous background. In later stages, patients develop telangiectasia, sebaceous hyperplasia, and rhinophyma.

Etiology

Rosacea is a follicular inflammatory disease for which the etiology remains uncertain. Unproven etiopathogenic theories are rife, including gastrointestinal infection with the "ulcer bacterium" *Helicobacter pylori*, immunologic reaction to *Demodex*

53

follicularum mites, abnormal responses to emotional stress, and unusual vascular reactions. The mainstay of treatment is antibiotics, suggesting that infection, or at least colonization, plays a significant role in the disease.

Rosacea patients are generally prone to flushing and blushing. This "flush and blush" reaction may occur spontaneously. Alternatively, it can be precipitated by factors such as emotional stress, heat, caffeine, sunlight, alcoholic beverages, and spicy foods. Rosacea occurs more commonly in fair-skinned individuals but can occur even in the darkest individuals. Rosacea is more common in women, but men are more prone to sebaceous hyperplasia, which may result in the disfiguring changes of rhinophyma. Rosacea occurs whether or not patients had significant amounts of acne in their earlier years.

Clinical Presentation

The hallmark of early rosacea is recurrent flushing and blushing of the face. Typically, the flushing and blushing are asymptomatic but highly embarassing. Patients may describe burning and irritation of the affected skin.

Figure 4-1

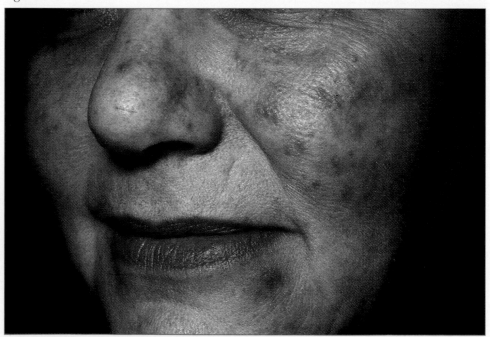

Striking erythema of the central face distinguishes rosacea from acne vulgaris.

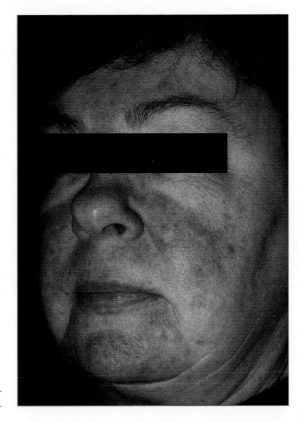

Figure 4-2

The nose and cheeks are the most commonly involved areas in rosacea patients.

The eruption of rosacea usually is localized to the central face but also may be found on the chest, neck, scalp, and back. The most common locations include the nose and the medial cheeks (Figs. 4-1 through 4-4). Erythema is common and may be accompanied by telangiectasias. As the eruption becomes more chronic, the development of telangiectasias becomes more prominent.

Recurrent crops of follicular inflammatory papules and pustules on a brightly erythematous base are a common feature. The erythema is far more than is expected with acne vulgaris, but the individual papules and pustules look acneiform. Lesions individually last for days to weeks, to be replaced by newer inflammatory lesions. Comedones, another feature of acne vulgaris, are notably absent.

In chronic roseacea, large inflammatory nodules, sebaceous hyperplasia, and connective tissue hyperplasia are dominant features. Fortunately, only a small proportion of these patients progress to these stages. Inflammatory nodules and tissue hyperplasia commonly affect the nose (rhinophyma) and cheeks. Eventually, the skin may become thickened and edematous, and this can be disfiguring.

A granulomatous type of rosacea exists that presents with infiltrative erythematous papules in a typical rosacea distribution. This granulomatous variant typically lacks the striking erythema and telangiectasia of typical rosacea.

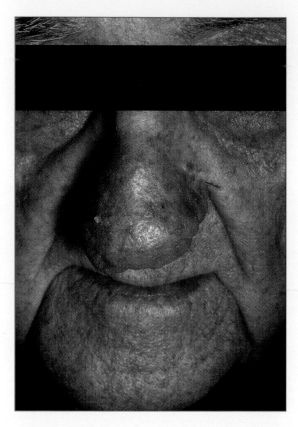

Figure 4-3

Early rhinophyma is becoming evident in this patient with chronic rosacea.

Twenty percent of rosacea patients may complain of mild ophthalmologic symptoms. Ophthalmologic involvement usually manifests as conjunctivitis or blepharitis and, more rarely, as iritis, episcleritis, or keratitis. Eye findings may be accompanied by pain or photophobia. Severe involvement may result in corneal opacities or blindness secondary to keratitis.

Evaluation of Patients

The diagnosis of rosacea is done clinically and rarely relies on laboratory testing. A history consistent with flushing and blushing reactions is helpful in confirming the diagnosis. It is not always possible for clinicians to differentiate rosacea from acne vulgaris (Table 4-1), but many of the treatments are similar. Rosacea tends to affect middle-aged and older adults, whereas acne vulgaris predominantly affects people in the second through fourth decades of life. If a diagnosis is difficult to

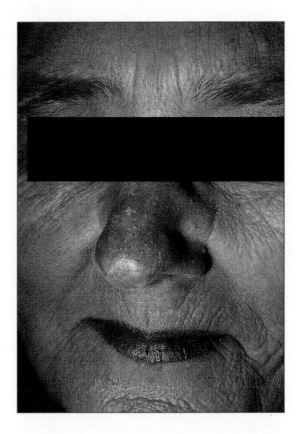

Figure 4-4

Rosacea limited to the nose.

make correctly, the clinician should consider referral to a dermatologist for another opinion. A skin biopsy specimen can be obtained for histopathologic evaluation if the clinician is unable to differentiate rosacea from other inflammatory facial conditions, but the authors have never needed to resort to this testing technique (Table 4-2).

Treatment

Rosacea is not curable but can be improved greatly with treatment. Clinicians should advise patients to avoid provoking stimuli such as sun exposure, hot beverages, and alcohol if any can be identified from the directed history. Minimal disease without ophthalmologic involvement may respond well to topical therapy alone. More severe disease or symptomatic ophthalmologic involvement should prompt the consideration of systemic management. With systemic therapy, better disease control

Table 4-1

Differentiating Rosacea from Acne

	ROSACEA	ACNE
Diffuse redness and/or telangiectasia	Common	Not usually present
Age >40	Common	Unusual
Comedones	Not present	Common
Eye irritation	Sometimes present	Not present
Pustules	Common	Common
Response to oral antibiotics	Common	Common

often is obtained by simultaneously using topical agents and systemic interventions.

Topical Therapy

The clinician should exercise care in treating rosacea patients with topical products because some patients have very sensitive skin. Harsh skin cleansing should be avoided. Topical corticosteroids may temporarily suppress inflammation but usually make rosacea worse over the long term. Accordingly, corticosteroid agents should be avoided.

Most topical agents are applied twice daily on the affected areas. Patients require 3 months of therapy for optimal dimunition in erythema, pustules, and papules. Ongoing therapy is required by many patients to help supress flares of the disease. Specific agents for therapy are discussed below.

METRONIDAZOLE

Metronidazole is available as a gel (Metrogel) or cream (Metrocream and Notitate) for topical use. All metronidazole products generally are well tolerated by patients, effective, and easy to apply. Occasionally, patients complain about irritation from any of these products. As with other topical antibiotics, treatment begins with twice-a-day use; once the disease is controlled, the frequency of application may be reduced to once a day or less to maintain control of the condition.

SULFACETAMIDE

Sulfacetamide is available in several topical formultions, including Sulfacet R, Klaron, and Novacet. These formulations are well tolerated by patients, effective, and easy to apply. They generally should not be administered to patients with hypersensitivity to sulfa antibiotics.

CLINDAMYCIN

Although not approved in the United States for rosacea, clindamycin gel and lotion (Cleocin) may be effective therapeutic agents for this disease. The gel and lotion preparations are water based and are well tolerated.

Table 4-2
Differential Diagnosis

Acne vulgaris	Typically has much less erythema and telangiectasia and may have comedones
Carcinoid syndrome	Results from release of vasoactive mediators from a malignant tumor; flushing atacks are paroxysmal, but other signs of rosacea, such as pustules and papules, are not seen
Contact dermatitis	Typically, scaling and/or minute vesicles are seen in irritant or allergic contact dermatitis; these features are absent in rosacea
Lupus erythematosus	Typically is photodistributed, and findings are often discovered in the ears and other locations; pustules are a rare component of the clinical picture, whereas in rosacea they are seen commonly
Seborrheic dermatitis	Although the central face may be involved, the nasolabial and melolabial folds are affected more commonly than is the nose, and often scaling and erythema are found in and around the ears, eyebrows, and scalp
Perioral dermatitis	Most commonly occurs in young women in a perioral distribution; also may occur in a perinasal or periocular distribution; typically responds well to rosacea treatments and may represent a form of rosacea

Systemic Therapy

More resistant or severe cases of rosacea should be treated with a systemic antibiotic agent. Any patient with ophthalmologic disease, regardless of the severity of the skin disease, also should be treated with an oral antibiotic. Systemic therapy usually is required over months to years. Patients can be treated with lower doses of systemic agents and can be weaned more quickly from those agents by using adjunctive topical therapy. However, tapering must be accomplished slowly over a period of months or the patient will be at risk for rebound disease flaring.

Specific agents appropriate for therapy are detailed below. While any of the antibiotics may be used as initial therapy, the choice is guided by the expense (tetracycline and erythromycin are relatively inexpensive), the potential for inconvenience (tetracyclines are better absorbed on an empty stomach), and side effects (erythromycin has a high propensity to cause gastrointestinal pain).

TETRACYCLINE

Tetracycline in doses of 250 to 500 mg twice daily can be effective in treating rosacea symptoms. Mild photosensitivity, yeast vaginitis, and nausea limit its use in some patients. This agent should be consumed 1 or more hours before eating or 2 hours after eating to ensure absorption.

DOXYCYCLINE (VIBRAMYCIN)

Doxycline in doses of 50 to 100 mg twice daily can be effective in treating rosacea symptoms. Extreme photosensitivity and yeast vaginitis limit its use in some patients.

MINOCYCLINE (MINOCIN)

Minocycline in doses of 50 to 100 mg twice daily can be effective in treating rosacea symptoms. Mild photosensitivity, yeast vaginitis, and hyperpigmentation limit its use in some patients.

OTHER ANTIBIOTIC AGENTS

Additional agents that ocasionally are helpful include erythromycin 500 to 1000 mg/d orally in divided doses and metronidazole (Flagyl) 500 mg/d orally in divided doses. Metronidalzole may interact with alcohol and may cause a disulfiram-like reaction. Accordingly, caution should be exercised in its use.

ISOTRETINOIN (ACCUTANE)

Isotretinoin treatment should be reserved for patients with severe involvement that has failed to respond to one or more antibiotic therapies. Isotretinoin in doses ranging from 0.5 to 2.0 mg/kg per day is most commonly used for a 16- to 20-week course. The more common side effects include headache, xerosis, cheilitis, conjunctivitis, epistaxis, gastrointestinal upset, myalgia, and arthralgia.

Isotretinoin is highly teratogenic, and reliable contraception for women of childbearing age is mandatory 1 month before therapy initiation and should continue until 1 month after therapy. The importance of effective birth control cannot be overemphasized, and a thorough informed consent should be obtained before beginning the medication. The clinician is strongly urged to follow the Pregnancy Prevention Program as outlined by the manufacturer. A negative pregnancy test should be obtained before the beginning of therapy and at monthly intervals during therapy. Isotretinoin is not mutagenic, and after discontinuation of the medication for 1 month, patients can safely conceive.

Laboratory monitoring for other side effects may vary with the clinician, but liver function and triglyceride monitoring should be done before the initiation of therapy and may be done as often as monthly thereafter.

Other Therapeutic Modalities

Telangiectasias and soft tissue hyperplasia are often resistant to systemic and topical antibiotic therapy, particularly when these changes have been present for a prolonged period. The 585-nm flash-lamp pulsed dye laser has been effective in treating telangiectasias. Several consecutive treatments may be necessary for resolution, depending on the degree of involvement. Soft tissue hyperplasia such as rhinophyma can be difficult to treat, and surgical modalities usually are required. Electrosurgery, carbon dioxide laser, and dermabrasion procedures sometimes are effective in improving the appearance of rhinophyma.

Prognosis

The long-term prognosis is variable. Generally, the pustular component of rosacea responds rapidly to treatment, while flushing and telangiectasia respond much more slowly. Once the pustules are well controlled, many patients maintain control with reduced doses of the oral agents or with topical products alone. While some patients may be able to discontinue therapy entirely (restarting it at the onset of a new flare), most patients require continued maintenance therapy to prevent immediate recurrence of the disease.

Bibliography

Dreizen S: The butterfly rash and the malar flush: What diseases do these signs reflect? *Postgrad Med* 89:225, 233, 1996.

Chalmers DA: Rosacea: Recognition and management for the primary care provider. *Nurse Pract* 22:23, 1997.

Chu T: Treatment of rosacea. *Practitioner* 237:941, 1993.

Jansen T, Plewig G: Rosacea: Classification and treatment. *J R Soc Med* 90:144, 1997.

Litt JZ: Rosacea: How to recognize and treat an age-related skin disease. *Geriatrics* 52:39, 1997.

Rebora A, Drago F, Parodi A: May *Helicobacter pylori* be important for dermatologists? *Dermatology* 191:6, 1995.

Shelley WB, Shelley ED, Burmeister V: Unilateral demodectic rosacea. *J Am Acad Dermatol* 20:915, 1989.

Smith KW: Perioral dermatitis with histopathologic features of granulomatous rosacea: Successful treatment with isotretinoin. *Cutis* 46:413, 1990.

Wilkin JK: Rosacea: Pathophysiology and treatment. *Arch Dermatol* 130:359, 1994.

Urticaria (Hives)

Background

Most patients with urticaria have short-lived idiopathic disease. Infections, drugs, foods, and contactants may be implicated in some patients. An unfortunate group of patients develops chronic urticaria or physical urticaria, which may last from months to decades. The mainstay of therapy is continuous histamine blockade, preferably with minimally sedating agents such as cetirizine, astemazole, and loratidine.

Clinical Features

In urticaria patients, one sees from a few to thousands of intensely itchy, short-lived wheals. The wheals consist of erythematous papules, plaques, arcs, and polycyclic forms with peripheral blanching (Figs. 5-1 through 5-6). Individual wheals last between 1 and 24 hours. Secondary changes, including excoriation and purpura, may be seen.

Risk Factors

Heredity may play a role in a small subset of urticaria patients. An autosomal dominant hereditary form of urticaria and/or angioedema results from C1 esterase inhibitor deficiency. Acquired C1 esterase deficiency has been noted in patients with malignancies and systemic lupus erythematosus. Specific subcategories of urticaria,

Figure 5-1

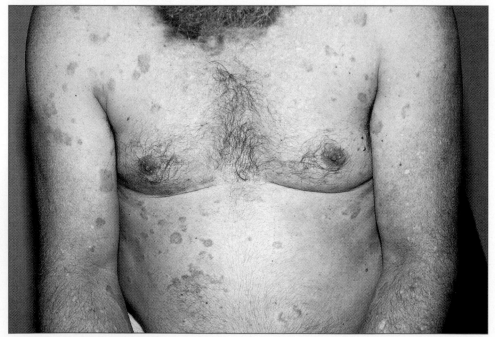

A patient with an acute eruption of urticaria.

Figure 5-2

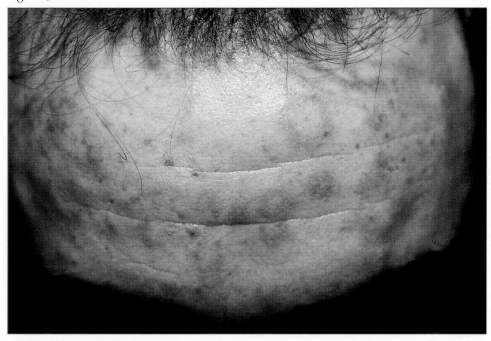

Annular and papular wheals.

including vibratory angioedema, heat urticaria, and cold-induced urticaria, have inherited forms.

Pathophysiology

The transudation of fluid from small cutaneous blood vessels results in urticarial lesions. The *peau d'orange* appearance results from this dermal edema. Mast cells play a primary role in this process. Mast cell granules contain histamine, chemotactic factors for eosinophils and neutrophils, prostaglandins, platelet-activating factor, and leukotrienes. All these products are released when a mast cell is stimulated. Histamine therefore is an important factor in the pathogenesis of urticaria. The type I IgE-mediated hypersensitivity state is a common immunologic mechanism involved in urticaria. Allergens involved in type I reactions may include medications and foods or result from infections and insect bites. Type III serum-sickness-like reactions sometimes are responsible for eliciting urticaria by activating the complement system. A large number of medications, including morphine, codeine, meperidine, quinine, aspirin, nonsteroidal anti-inflammatory agents, and

Figure 5-3

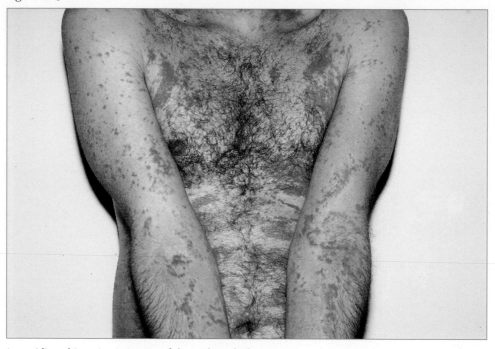

Acute idiopathic urticaria in one of the authors (AF).

radiocontrast media, directly stimulate histamine release. Specific physical promoters, including cold, heat, vibration, and light, result in histamine and other mediator release in predisposed individuals.

Types of Urticaria

Acute Urticaria

The abrupt onset of one to hundreds of spontaneous wheals which may be associated with dermatographism is characteristic of urticaria. This usually clears in 1 to 6 weeks. The etiology is occasionally identified.

Chronic Urticaria

Typical short-lived urticarial wheals last for months to decades. The natural history suggests that 50 percent resolve in the first 6 months, perhaps because of an auto-

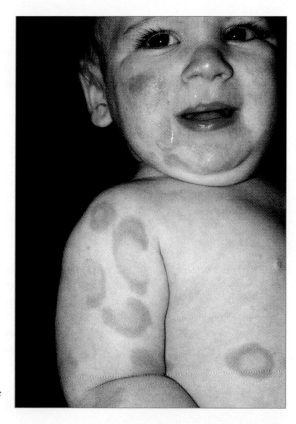

Figure 5-4

Acute idiopathic urticaria in one of the author's (SF) children.

antibody directed at the mast cell IgE receptor. Circulating levels of a single anti-mast cell IgE receptor antibody are relevant to the pathogenesis of severe chronic urticaria in about 25 percent of patients. Other autoantibodies may explain chronic urticaria in other patients, but clinical tests for those autoantibodies are not available. Other identifiable factors that should be considered include chronic infections, drug exposures, and food allergies. It is rare for exposure to a single allergen to explain chronic urticaria.

Adrenergic Urticaria

Adrenergic urticaria is a rare but distinct reported condition in which lesions develop during phases of stress. Attacks are associated with an increase in the plasma concentrations of noradrenaline, adrenaline, prolactin, and dopamine. The symptoms can be reproduced by the intradermal injection of adrenaline and noradrenaline. This condition can be treated successfully with the ß-adrenergic blocker propanolol. Other ß-adrenergic blockers also may be effective.

Physical Urticaria

Skin trauma causes mast cells to release histamine and causes a wheal at the site of trauma. A variety of precipitating factors may induce the disease in different patients (Table 5-1). Patients may present with more than one type of physical urticaria (e.g., heat and cold urticaria).

Some types, such as aquagenic, cholinergic, and cold urticaria, may be associated with angioedema, wheezing, and hypotension. Treatment consists of minimizing the offending stimulus. The clinical response to antihistaminic agents is variable. Patients with symptomatic dermatographism may be difficult to diagnose, unless they have recently scratched or the clinician performs a physical dermatographic challenge. Analogous situations apply to most of the physical urticarial conditions.

Angioedema

Virtually any type of urticaria may be seen in conjunction with angioedema, or angioedema may exist as a singular entity. Mucous membrane edema may be associated with uricarial wheals on the skin. Angioedema may be life-threatening as a result of respiratory compromise and anaphylactic shock. The same idiopathic, drug, food, and physical agents that cause other forms of urticaria may cause angioedema. If it is recurrent and severe, angioedema may extremely rarely be

Figure 5-5

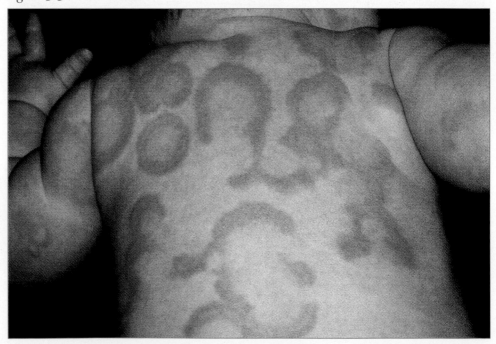

Acute idiopathic urticaria in one of the author's (SF) children.

Table 5-1
Physical Urticaria

Type	Precipitating Factors	Reaction Time	Duration	Diagnostic Test	Reported Effective Treatments
Symptomatic dermatographism	Stroking or rubbing skin	Minutes	2–3 h	Gentle stroking uninvolved skin	Antihistamines
Pressure urticaria	Pressure	3–12 h	8–24 h	Pressure challenge on shoulder of 7 kg for 15 min	Topical corticosteroids, sulfasalazine, dapsone, and cetirizine
Solar urticaria	Ultraviolet	2–5 min	15 min–3 h	Phototesting	Sunscreens, chloroquine, ß-carotene, phototherapy, astemizole, terfenidine, cetirizine, doxepin, plasmapheresis
Cold urticaria	Low temperature	2–5 min or up to 3 h	1–2 h or up tp 48 h	Ice cube to skin for 20 min	Cold desensitization, antihistamines such as cyproheptadine and doxepin, ketotifen, terbutaline with aminophylline
Heat urticaria	High temperature	2–5 min	1 h	Warming of the affected part, e.g., to 43°C for 5 min	Desensitization by repeated exposure to local heat, antihistamines such as astemazole and doxepin
Cholinergic urticaria	Physical exercise, sweating, hot baths	2–5 min	30–60 min	Exercise or hot bath provocation	Antihistamines, ketotifen, or cold water to sweating skin
Aquagenic urticaria	Contact with water	Up to 30 min	Hours	Water compresses at 35–36°C to back for 10 min	Antihistamines, phototherapy
Vibration urticaria	Vibration	2–5 min	60 min	Application of kitchen mixer to forearm	Avoidance of stimuli

Source: Modified from Jorizzo JL, Smith EB: The physical urticarias: An update and review. *Arch Dermatol* 118:194, 1982

Figure 5-6

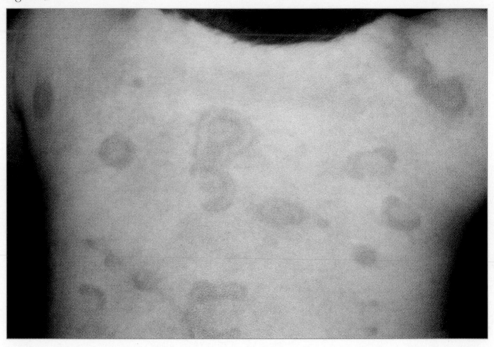

Acute idiopathic uriticaria in one of the author's (SF) children.

associated with C1 esterase inhibitor deficiency. Anaphylaxis may be recurrent and life-threatening, and patients who experience this reaction pattern should be treated acutely with systemic corticosteroid agents, antihistamines, and epinephrine. Self-injecting epinephrine kits may be lifesaving in patients with severe angioedema, and counseling about their appropriate use is indicated.

Contact Urticaria

Contact with a specific allergen causes histamine release at the contact site, with associated itching, redness, and wheals. Not all patients have visible disease. Lesions begin within 30 min of contact and are limited to areas of direct contact. Common urticarial contact allergens include rubber, cinnamic aldehyde, and sorbic and benzoic acids. These allergens may be present in clothing, cosmetics, and toiletries, and there may be occupational exposures. Atopic patients may be more prone to develop this condition. The most important aspect of treatment in this type of urticaria is avoidance of the allergen.

Contact urticaria has been reported in different patients to result from direct skin contact with numerous items; some of the more interesting items include semen, spices, cornstarch, globe artichoke, litchi fruit, kiwi fruit, watermelon, shiitake mushrooms, rice, buckwheat flour, mold on salami casing, nickel, beef, cow milk, pork, fish, dog saliva, tobacco, locusts, and mouse hair.

Evaluation of a Patient with Urticaria

Overview

Aside from the physical urticarial diseases, the etiology is not commonly discerned. History helps identify the type of urticaria, helps eliminate nonurticarial diseases, and may help identify the cause of eruption. Extensive laboratory evaluation is rarely indicated, except when the history suggests that a chronic infection or another systemic cause may be contributory. The clinician should focus on the history: Patients with urticaria are distressed and under duress; they may recall unrelated exposures from earlier decades and neglect antibiotic therapy instituted a few days earlier (Fig. 5-7).

Duration and Prior History

When did *this* episode start? Has anything like this happened to you before? These questions help determine whether there is an acute or chronic process. If previous episodes have occurred, this question may help identify the precipitating factors.

Figure 5-7

In all patients
    Directed history and physical examination

In selected patients
    Occasionally helpful tests
        Complete blood count with differential analysis
        Erythrocyte sedimentation rate
    Rarely helpful tests
        Antinuclear antibody
        Blood chemistry profile
        CH_{50}
        Cryoproteins
        Hepatitis B and C virus surface antigen and antibody
        Radioallergosorbent test for specific IgE
        Skin tests for IgE-mediated reactions
        Stool examination for ova and parasites

Diagnostic algorithm for urticaria.

Location

Where are the spots typically located? Urticaria limited to the hands and forearms or another localized area may suggest contact urticaria. Physical urticarias tend to have limited rather than generalized distributions.

Recent Infections

Have you been ill in the past several weeks? The onset of urticaria may occur from minutes to weeks after the precipitating event. Infections of the following types may precipitate urticaria:

- Bacterial: focal sepsis, including sinusitis, pharyngitis, and urinary tract infections
- Viral: respiratory infections and hepatitis
- Fungal: vaginal candidiasis
- Parasitic: protozoal and helminthic infections

Drugs

Have you started taking new medications in the past month? Have you taken any antibiotics? Virtually any medication can cause urticaria, but antibiotics are particularly likely causes. It is unclear whether antibiotics are a common cause because they are commonly used or whether they have a marked predisposition to producing urticaria. The clinician should look for a good temporal history; often, urticarial drug eruptions begin shortly after the introduction of a medication. Discontinuation of the medication may not result in immediate cessation of the eruption; urticaria may persist for weeks. In a patient in whom antibiotics are suspected offenders, one must remember that focal infections also can cause urticaria. Histamine-releasing drugs that can immediately precipitate urticaria (or angioedema) include atropine, codeine, curare, dextran, hydralazine, morphine, pentamidine, and radiocontrast media. Aspirin and nonsteroidal anti-inflammatory agents may precipitate urticaria through other mechanisms or exacerbate existing urticaria.

Foods

Do your hives start after you eat specific foods? Foods are an uncommon cause of urticaria. Acute or recurrent attacks occur within minutes or hours of ingestion and last for hours to days. The main foods implicated in urticaria are eggs, nuts, chocolate, fish and shellfish, tomatoes, pork, strawberries, milk, cheese, spices, yeast, and preservatives.

Contactants

Do your hives begin after you wear rubber gloves or other clothing or when you come in contact with anything in particular? Contact urticaria usually has a rapid onset after exposure; patients may easily make this association.

Laboratory Evaluation

In acute urticaria, a self-limited disease, laboratory evaluation is not needed. In chronic urticaria, laboratory studies are more commonly useful for psychological rather than medical reasons. If testing is required, consider the following:

- Complete blood count with differential. Examine for evidence of eosinophilia, as eosinophilia may indicate a parasitic infection that requires further evaluation.
- Erythrocyte sedimentation rate (ESR). If it is normal or extremely elevated, this may be helpful. Extremely high ESRs indicate chronic inflammation that requires further evaluation.
- Multichemistry panel. Examine for evidence of abnormal protein levels or hepatic and renal dysfunction.
- Throat culture for streptococcal infection. When other symptoms and signs suggest that this may be contributory.
- Urinalysis. Examine for evidence of urinary tract infection.
- Stool examination for ova and parasites. This is rarely helpful, but virtually any form of intestinal or other parasitosis may induce urticaria.
- Radioallergenosorbent tests (RAST). These tests may help identify specific allergies to foods and drugs. Positive results are frequently irrelevant, and in the vast majority of patients these tests bear no fruitful results. These tests are appropriate only in patients who have failed to respond to a broad range of therapeutic interventions in chronic urticaria.
- Prick and scratch testing. The cost-effectiveness and diagnostic value of these tests have never been assessed accurately. In select patients these techniques may have value; the vast majority of patients derive no benefit from their use. These tests are appropriate only in patients who have failed to respond to a broad range of therapeutic interventions for chronic urticaria. These tests should be performed only by experienced clinicians, as interpretation of the results requires clinical skill and severe reactions are possible.

Therapy

Overview

The mainstay of urticaria therapy remains long-acting antihistaminic treatment with agents such as loratadine and cetirazine (Fig. 5-8). If sedating antihistamines such as diphenhydramine and hydroxyzine are used, they are best administered at bedtime. If systemic corticosteroids must be used, the duration of therapy generally should be limited to less than 1 week. Even if it is not thought to be directly related to the current eruption, the use of aspirin, nonsteroidal anti-inflammatory agents, opiate agents, and other known exacerbators of urticaria should be discontinued.

Figure 5-8

Identify and remove precipitating factors when possible	
Administer long-acting H$_1$ antihistaminic agents in doses sufficient to improve symptoms; required doses may be many times the indicated dosage	
If disease is uncontrolled, consider addition of secondary agents to H$_1$ antihistaminic agents	Systemic corticosteroid agents are rarely appropriate for long-term use
	H$_2$ antihistaminic agents in combination with H$_1$ antihistaminic agents
	Anti-inflammatory agents demonstrated to have value in treating chronic urticaria (e.g., dapsone, cyclosporine, methotrexate)
Consider elimination diets	

Therapeutic algorithm for urticaria.

Antihistaminic Agents

Because of patient compliance, long-acting, minimally sedating antihistamine agents such as astemazole (Hismanal), cetirizine (Zyrtec), fexofenadine (Allegra), and loratidine (Claritin) are more effective than short-acting agents (Table 5-2). Loratidine has little sedation even in doses up to 40 mg/d, high efficacy, and excellent patient acceptance. Cetizine is also an effective agent, but its efficacy is limited by sedation that becomes particularly evident in doses of 20 to 40 mg/d in adults. Both loratadine and cetirazine are safe, patients often require treatment in higher than recommended doses, and neither agent has significant drug interactions. Astemazole is a useful antihistaminic agent with an extremely long half-life but has numerous potentially life-threatening drug interactions. Astemazole is not safe at higher than recommended doses and is the most cardiotoxic antihistaminic agent marketed.

Fexofenadine may be the least effective of this group of antihistaminic agents, but it lacks the sedation and medication interactions of its parent compound terfenadine (Seldane). As with terfenadine, preliminary evidence suggests that fexofenadine may promote cardiac arrhythmias. Unless comparative studies are published that show the superiority of fexofenadine over other antihistaminic agents, we will continue to reserve judgment on its safety and efficacy.

Although quite sedating and requiring thrice-daily dosing, hydroxyzine has mild anxiolytic activity and may be particularly useful in distressed urticaria patients at night. Diphenhydramine may play a similar role and is best used at bedtime. A cost-effective option for good 24-h histamine blockade is to use a nonsedating antihistamine in the morning and a sedating antihistamine at bedtime.

Astemazole and doxepin are antihistaminic antidepressant agents. These agents require the longest time to achieve pharmacologic steady state, but histamine blockade is the most prolonged. Doxepin has the most side effects of any of these agents

Table 5-2

Select H$_1$ Antihistaminic Agents

ANTIHISTAMINIC	INITIAL ADULT DAILY DOSE (MG*)	DOSING INTERVAL, H	HISTAMINE BLOCKADE	SIDE EFFECT PROFILE
Acrivastine	8	6–8	++[†]	+
Amitriptyline	10–100	24	++++	++++
Astemazole	10	24	+++	+
Cetirizine	10	24	+++	+
Chlorpheniramine	4	4–6	++	+
Clemastine	1	12	++	++
Cyproheptadine	4	8	+	+
Diphenhydramine	25–50	6–8	+	+++
Doxepin	10–100	24	++++	++++
Fexofenadine	60–120	12	++	+
Hydroxyzine	10–25	6–8	+++	++
Loratidine	10	24	+++	+
Promethazine	12.5–25	6–12	+++	+++

* For agents that are noncardiotoxic, patients may require much higher doses to control symptoms.
† + = little; ++++ = maximal.

but may be the most potent and has the longest duration. It is unclear that either astemazole and doxepin is more effective in urticaria than are older antihistaminic agents such as hydroxyzine.

The sedative effects of sedating antihistaminic agents are potentiated by benzodiazepines, other neuropsychiatric agents, and alcohol. Anticholinergic side effects such as xerostomia, urinary retention, and impotence are more common with less specific older agents and antihistamine-like agents such as amitriptyline and doxepin. Some patients, particularly children, paradoxically are stimulated by sedating drugs. Rare side effects include seizures, weight gain, and anaphylaxis. Although these medications are not contraindicated, special precautions should be exercised in those operating heavy machinery and those with sicca syndrome, epilepsy, prostatic hypertrophy, glaucoma, and porphyria.

Fatal cardiac arrhythmias can occur when astemazole and terfenadine interact with macrolide antibiotics, including erythromycin and clarithromycin, and systemic antifungal agents, including fluconazole, itraconazole, and ketoconazole, and these agents also interact with cisapride and lovostatin. Among the nonsedating agents, loratidine, cetirizine, and fexofenadine have few if any known significant drug interactions.

Antihistaminic agents may be one of the safest classes of agents to use during pregnancy. Nevertheless, whenever possible, it is prudent to avoid all unnecessary agents. Chlorpheniramine, diphenhydramine, and hydroxyzine generally are considered safe during pregnancy.

H_2 Antihistamines

Modest evidence supports the occasional use of H_2 antihistamines in treating urticaria. Monotherapy with H_2 blockers has minimal efficacy, but cimetidine may increase plasma concentrations of H_1 antihistamines. In urticaria, H_1 antihistamines such as chlorpheniramine may be combined with agents such as cimetidine and ranitidine to enhance the therapeutic effect, and H_2 agents decrease itching and whealing. No published study has analyzed the addition of H_2 agents to the more efficacious newer antihistamines astemazole, cetirizine, and loratidine. Accordingly, at best these agents should be considered secondary treatments when high doses of H_1 antihistamines have failed. An example of dosing is ranitidine 300 mg bid.

Corticosteroid Use in Urticaria

In a controlled trial, prednisone 20 mg every 12 h for 4 days combined with hydroxyzine was more effective than hydroxyzine alone in relieving itching and rash. The problem with this study is that it used a short-acting antihistaminic agent, hydroxyzine. Nevertheless, corticosteroids are likely to be effective in achieving rapid control of acute urticaria. When one initiates systemic corticosteroid treatment, simultaneously initiating adequate doses of long-acting antihistaminic therapy can help provide better control. Although effective, single-dose-per-day schedules of a short-acting corticosteroid agent such as prednisone (or an equivalent) may not provide 24-h blockade of symptoms. We give doses of 0.5 mg/kg of prednisone for 1 week. Because of the significant side effect profile, long-term systemic corticosteroid agents in chronic urticaria may constitute effective treatment but rarely are used as a first choice.

Other Therapeutic Approaches toward Urticaria

Combinations of H_1 Blockers

Consider combining minimally sedating antihistamines such as cetirizine, loratidine, and astemazole with a sedating antihistamine. As was noted above, excellent choices include bedtime doses of hydroxyzine, chlorpheniramine, and doxepin.

Elimination Diets

If food is thought to be implicated and the patient is highly motivated, this modality may be employed. Eliminate all foods except chicken and rice with no spices, preservatives, or condiments. After 1 week add one simple food, a single spice, or a single food additive per day. If the urticaria continues unabated after several weeks, food is unlikely to be contributory.

Dapsone

Dapsone is an anti-inflammatory and antineutrophilic agent that may benefit some patients with recalcitrant urticaria. This agent is particularly beneficial in urticarial vasculitis, a related condition. The dose that is typically required is 50 to 100 mg/d in adults.

UVB and PUVA

Ultraviolet B (UVB) light or psoralen with ultraviolet A photochemotherapy (PUVA) can be helpful in select patients with recalcitrant disease. Once therapeutic results have been achieved after 15 to 20 treatments, maintenance therapy often is required. Chronic urticaria, solar urticaria, and symptomatic dermatographism are reported to be improved with phototherapy.

Antibiotics

Under the hypothesis that chronic antigen stimulation promotes urticaria, treatment with an empirical course of broad-spectrum antibiotics and/or antifungal agents has anecdotal support. Despite a lack of controlled trials demonstrating efficacy, this approach may be employed with limited success.

Epinephrine

Epinephrine is used in emergency departments and occasionally on outpatients to control respiratory symptoms. Patients with a history of airway obstruction should be prescribed an epinephrine injection device (e.g., Anakit, Epipen) to allow them to overcome acute airway obstruction. All patients requiring epinephrine injection should be evaluated immediately by a physician. Oral epinephrine is rarely indicated because of its numerous undesirable side effects.

Topical Agents

Although traditionally thought to play a minimal therapeutic role, oxatomide gel and dechlorpheniramine cream have been shown to decrease itching and erythema. They are not currently available in the United States. Topical clobetasol may decrease symptomatic dermatographism, but this agent is unlikely to be beneficial for this use. For extremely limited disease, topical agents may prove beneficial.

Miscellaneous Therapies

The following therapies have been found to be effective:

Cyclosporin A
Danazol
Intravenous immunoglobulin (IVIG)
Methotrexate
Nifedipine
Relaxation therapy
Stanozolol.

Bibliography

Barlow RJ, Macdonald DM, Black AK, Greaves MW: The effects of topical corticosteroids on delayed pressure urticaria. *Arch Dermatol Res* 287:285, 1995.

Beltrani VS: Urticaria and angioedema. *Dermatol Clin* 14:171, 1996.

Bleehen SS, Thomas SE, Greaves MW, et al: Cimetidine and chlorpheniramine in the treatment of chronic idiopathic urticaria: A multi-centre randomized double-blind study. *Br J Dermatol* 117:81, 1987.

Bressler RB, Sowell K, Huston DP: Therapy of chronic idiopathic urticaria with nifedipine: Demonstration of beneficial effect in a double-blinded, placebo-controlled, crossover trial. *J Allergy Clin Immunol* 83:756, 1989.

Brestel EP, Thrush LB: The treatment of glucocorticosteroid-dependent chronic urticaria with stanozolol. *J Allergy Clin Immunol* 82:265, 1998.

Czarnetzki BM: *Urticaria.* Berlin, Springer-Verlag, 1986.

Dayani A, Gould DJ, Campbell S: Delayed pressure urticaria: Treatment with dapsone. *J Dermatol Treat* 3:61, 1992.

Duke WW: Urticaria caused specifically by action of physical agents. *JAMA* 83:3, 1924.

Engler RJ, Squire E, Benson P: Chronic sulfasalazine therapy in the treatment of delayed pressure urticaria and angioedema. *Ann Allergy Asthma Immunol* 74:155, 1995.

Farnam J, Grant JA, Guernsey BG, et al: Successful treatment of chronic idiopathic urticaria and angioedema with cimetidine alone. *J Allergy Clin Immunol* 73:842, 1984.

Fradin MS, Ellis CN, Goldfarb MT, et al: Oral cyclosporin for severe chronic idiopathic urticaria and angioedema. *J Am Acad Dermatol* 25:1065, 1991.

Grattan CE, Francis DM, Hide M, Greaves MW: Detection of circulating histamine releasing autoantibodies with functional properties of anti-IgE in chronic urticaria. *Clin Exp Allergy* 21:695, 1991.

Greaves MW: The physical urticarias. *Clin Exp Allergy* 21 (suppl 1):284, 1991.

Hannuksela M, Haahtela T: Hypersensitivity reactions to food additives. *Allergy* 42:561, 1987.

Haustein UF: Adrenergic urticaria and adrenergic pruritus. *Acta Dermato Venereol* 70:82, 1990.

Heese A, van Hintzenstern J, Peters KP, et al: Allergic and irritant reactions to rubber gloves in medical health services: Spectrum, diagnostic approach, and therapy. *J Am Acad Dermatol* 25:831, 1991.

Hide M, Francis DM, Grattan CE, et al: The pathogenesis of chronic idiopathic urticaria: New evidence suggests an auto-immune basis and implications for treatment. *Clin Exp Allergy* 24:624, 1994.

Higgins EM, Friedmann PS: Clinical report and investigation of a patient with localized heat urticaria. *Acta Dermato Venereol* 71:434, 1991.

Huston DP, Bressler RB, Kaliner M, et al: Prevention of mast-cell degranulation by ketotifen in patients with physical urticarias. *Ann Intern Med* 104:507, 1986.

Husz S, Toth-Kasa I, Kiss M, Dobozy A: Treatment of cold urticaria. *Int J Dermatol* 33:210, 1994.

Jaffer AM: Sulfasalazine in the treatment of corticosteroid-dependent chronic idiopathic urticaria. *J Allergy Clin Immunol* 88:964, 1991.

Jancelewicz Z: Controlled trial of H1 antagonists in the treatment of chronic idiopathic urticaria. *Ann Allergy* 67:433, 1991.

Johnsson M, Falk ES, Volden G: UVB treatment of factitious urticaria. *Photo Dermatol* 4:302, 1987.

Jorizzo JL, Smith EB: The physical urticarias: An update and review. *Arch Dermatol* 118:194, 1982.

Kemp AS, Schembri G: An elimination diet for chronic urticaria of childhood. *Med J Aust* 143:234, 1985.

Kennard CD, Ellis CN: Pharmacologic therapy for urticaria. *J Am Acad Dermatol* 25:176, 1991.

Kligman AM: The spectrum of contact urticaria. Wheals, erythema, and pruritus. *Dermatol Clin* 8:57, 1990.

Kobza Black A, Greaves MW, Champion RH, Pye RJ: The urticarias 1990. *Br J Dermatol* 124:100, 1991.

Lawlor F, Black AK, Murdoch RD, Greaves MW: Symptomatic dermographism: Wealing, mast cells and histamine are decreased in the skin following long-term application of a potent topical corticosteroid. *Br J Dermatol* 121:629, 1989.

Leenutaphong V, Holzle E, Plewig G, et al: Plasmapheresis in solar urticaria. *Dermatologica* 182:35, 1991.

Leigh IM, Ramsay CA: Localised heat urticaria treated by inducing tolerance to heat. *Br J Dermatol* 92:191, 1975.

Lewis J, Lieberman P, Treadwell G, Erffmeyer J: Exercise-induced urticaria, angioedema, and anaphylactoid episodes. *J Allergy Clin Immunol* 68:432, 1981.

Locci F, Del Giacco GS: Treatment of chronic idiopathic urticaria with topical preparations: Controlled study of oxatomide gel versus dechlorpheniramine cream. *Drugs Exp Clin Res* 17:399, 1991.

Logan RA, O'Brian TJ, Greaves MW: The effect of psoralen photochemotherapy (PUVA) on symptomatic dermatographism. *Clin Exp Dermatol* 14:25, 1989.

Markham A, Wagstaff AJ: Fexofenadine. *Drugs* 55:269, 1998.

Moscati RM, Moore GP: Comparison of cimetidine and diphenhydramine in the treatment of acute urticaria. *Ann Emerg Med* 19:12, 1990.

Neittaanmaki H, Fraki JE: Combination of localized heat urticaria and cold urticaria. Release of histamine in suction blisters and successful treatment of heat urticaria with doxepin. *Clin Exp Dermatol* 13:87, 1988.

Neittaanmaki H, Jaaskelainen T, Harvima RJ, Fraki JE: Solar urticaria: Demonstration of histamine release and effective treatment with doxepin. *Photo Dermatol* 6:52, 1989.

Neittaanmaki H, Myohanen T, Fraki JE: Comparison of cinnarizine, cyproheptadine, doxepin, and hydroxyzine in treatment of idiopathic cold urticaria: Usefulness of doxepin. *J Am Acad Dermatol* 11:483, 1984.

Niimi N, Francis DM, Kermani F, et al: Dermal mast cell activation by autoantibodies against the high affinity IgE receptor in chronic urticaria. *J Invest Dermatol* 106:1001, 1996.

O'Donnel BF, Barlow RJ, Kobza Black A, et al: Response of severe chronic urticaria to intravenous immunoglobulin (IVIG). *Br J Dermatol* 131 (suppl 44):23, 1994.

Olafsson JH, Larko O, Roupe G, et al: Treatment of chronic urticaria with PUVA or UVA plus placebo: A double-blind study. *Arch Dermatol Res* 278:228, 1986.

Ormerod AD: Urticaria: Recognition, causes and treatment. *Drugs* 48:717, 1994.

Panconesi E, Lotti T: Aquagenic urticaria. *Clin Dermatol* 5:49, 1987.

Parker RK, Crowe MJ, Guin JD: Aquagenic urticaria. *Cutis* 50:283, 1992.

Paul E, Bodeker RH: Treatment of chronic urticaria with terfenadine and ranitidine: A randomized double-blind study in 45 patients. *Eur J Clin Pharmacol* 31:277, 1986.

Pola J, Subiza J, Armentia A, et al: Urticaria caused by caffeine. *Ann Allergy* 60:207, 1988.

Pollack CV Jr, Romano TJ: Outpatient management of acute urticaria: The role of prednisone. *Ann Emerg Med* 26:547, 1995.

Sabroe RA, Francis DM, Barr RM, et al: Anti-Fc(epsilon)RI auto antibodies and basophil histamine releasability in chronic idiopathic urticaria. *J Allergy Clin Immunol* 102:651, 1998.

Salo OP, Kauppinen K, Mannisto PT: Cimetidine increases the plasma concentration of hydroxyzine. *Acta Dermato-Venereologica* 66:349, 1986.

Shertzer CL, Lookingbill DP: Effects of relaxation therapy and hypnotizability in chronic urticaria. *Arch Dermatol* 123:913, 1987.

Stafford CT: Urticaria as a sign of systemic disease. *Ann Allergy* 64:264, 1990.

Tanphaichitr K: Chronic urticaria associated with bacterial infection. *Cutis* 27:653, 1981.

Tharp MD: Chronic urticaria: Pathophysiology and treatment approaches. *J Allergy Clin Immunol* 98:S325, 1996.

Weiner MJ: Methotrexate in corticosteroid-resistant urticaria. *Ann Intern Med* 110:848, 1989.

Wong E, Eftekhari N, Greaves MW, et al: Beneficial effects of danazol on symptoms and laboratory changes in cholinergic urticaria. *Br J Dermatol* 116:553, 1987.

Zuraw BL: Urticaria, angioedema, and autoimmunity. *Clin Lab Med* 17:559, 1997.

Infectious Skin Diseases

Chapter 6

Cutaneous and Mucosal Candidiasis

Background

Infections of cutaneous and mucosal epithelium by *Candida* spp. occur in all age groups and have a wide range of clinical presentations. Most candidal infections are caused by *Candida albicans,* an opportunistic yeastlike fungus. Other species sometimes are isolated from cultures of infected areas, including *Torulopsis glabrata* and *C. tropicalis.* The oral and genital mucosa, intertriginous body folds, diaper area, and paronychium are the most commonly affected clinical sites.

Etiology

Candida spp. may colonize the oropharynx, gastrointestinal tract, and vagina of some normal individuals. *Candida* never inhabits the normal keratinized skin surface. A combination of many factors may cause these normally commensal candidal organisms to become pathogenic and infect keratinized skin. Colonization is aided by local factors, including heat, occlusion, moisture, friction, and loss of epithelial barrier function. Many other factors, such as systemic disease (diabetes mellitus, hypothyroidism, malnutrition, renal failure), immunodeficiency states [acquired immune deficiency syndrome (AIDS), immunosuppressive agents, malignancy], and antimicrobial agents, predispose individuals to develop candidiasis. Changes in the microflora resulting from any or all of these factors predispose susceptible individuals toward candidiasis. It is not known why some women, for instance, always develop vaginal candidiasis after the administration of antibiotics whereas other women never develop these infections. Individual susceptibility may play a larger role than is appreciated. Candidal infections range in severity from benign and superficial to systemic and fatal.

Clinical Presentation

Oral Candidiasis

Oral candidiasis presents clinically in several different forms. Pseudomembranous candidiasis (thrush), which manifests as white patches affecting the tongue, buc-

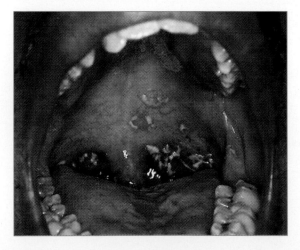

Figure 6-1

Thrush with characteristic patches on the palate. (From Freedberg I et al, eds: *Dermatology in General Medicine, 5th ed.* New York, McGraw-Hill, 1993, p. 2361.)

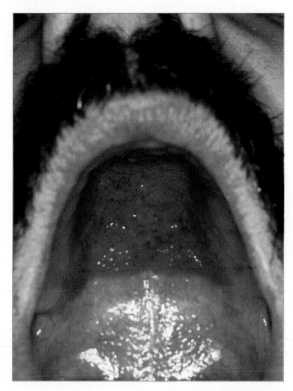

Figure 6-2

Acute atrophic candidiasis under dentures. (From Freedberg I et al, eds: *Dermatology in General Medicine, 5th ed.* New York, McGraw-Hill, 1993, p. 2361.)

cal mucosa, palate, and oropharynx, is the most common presentation (Fig. 6-1). The white patches tend to bleed easily when scraped gently with a tongue blade. Curdlike material reminiscent of cottage cheese can be removed easily with a tongue blade. Thrush develops most commonly in young children and older adults. The clinician should inquire about recent predisposing factors such as diabetes mellitus and recent antimicrobial therapy. In the absence of these factors, oral candidiasis may be a harbinger of an underlying immunodeficiency state, especially humman immunodefieciency virus (HIV), or a malignancy.

Acute Atrophic Candidiasis

Acute atrophic candidiasis presents as painful, atrophic erythematous plaques on the dorsum of the tongue or gums (see Fig. 6-2). Systemic antimicrobial therapy or corticosteroid metered-dose inhalant therapy may predispose a patient to candidal glossitis.

Dental Stomatitis

Denture stomatitis occurs when dental appliances come into contact with the oral mucosa and presents as sharply delineated mucosal edema and erythema. Poorly fitted dentures and dentures worn for long periods of time put a patient at risk of developing denture stomatitis. Many patients are reluctant to replace older dentures and chronically suffer from dental stomatitis.

Angular Cheilitis

Erythematous, fissured plaques arising on the oral commissures suggest a diagnosis of angular cheilitis (Fig. 6-3). Angular cheilitis may be a primary phenomenon or can occur in association with thrush or denture stomatitis. Angular cheilitis is most common in edentulous individuals.

Median Rhomboid Glossitis

Median rhomboid glossitis is a rare chronic candidal infection that creates papillary atrophy of the posterior dorsal tongue. Any oral candidal infection can lead to pain and burning of the mouth or odynophagia.

Candidal Vulvovaginitis

Candidal vulvovaginitis manifests as erythematous white plaques on the genital mucosa. Satellite pustules or erythematous scaling plaques also may be found on the adjacent vulva or scrotum. Candidal vaginitis often produces a creamy white discharge and is found more commonly in women who are pregnant, are taking oral contraceptives, or are immunocompromised. Pruritus, burning, and pain often are prominent symptoms. It is important to distinguish yeast infections from bacterial vaginosis, trichomonas infections, and other sexually transmitted diseases.

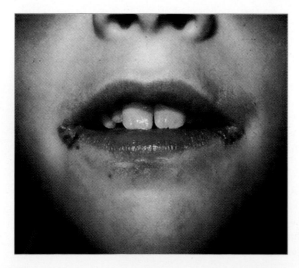

Figure 6-3

Perlèche with erythema and fissuring at the corners of the mouth. (From Weinberg S et al.: *Color Atlas of Pediatric Dermatology,* New York, McGraw-Hill, 1999, p. 580.)

Figure 6-4

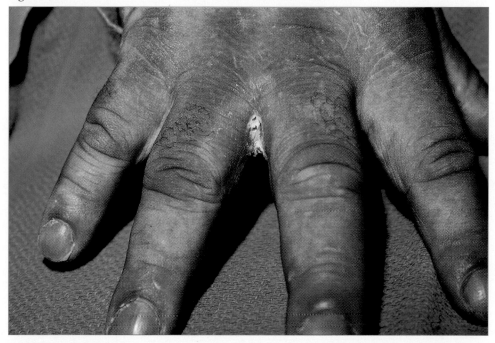

Moist, macerated skin on an erythematous base in the finger web spaces is typical of candidiasis.

Candidal Balanitis

Candidal balanitis is most commonly seen in men with diabetes mellitus. Candidal balanitis is likely to produce erythema and vesiculopustules on the glans penis but may spread to other portions of the penis. It is found more commonly in uncircumcised men.

Cutaneous Candidiasis

The most common form of cutaneous candidiasis is intertriginous candidiasis. Candidal intertrigo presents in the intertriginous surfaces of the inguinal, perineal, inframammary, and finger web spaces, where occlusion, heat, and moisture are major factors (Fig. 6-4). Irritant contact dermatitis often plays a major role in the development of intertrigo. Intertrigo appears as macerated, erythematous plaques with peripheral scaling and may feature satellite pustules and ulcerations. Obesity, diabetes mellitus, and systemic antibiotics are predisposing factors for intertrigo. Diaper dermatitis is a variant of intertrigo found in the diaper area in children; it is caused by the same factors of occlusion, heat, moisture, and irritation (Fig. 6-5).

Figure 6-5

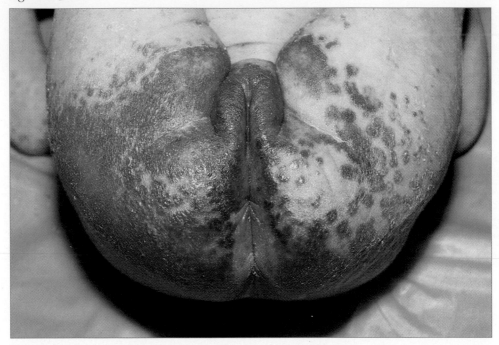

Diaper rashes may be complicated by abundant overgrowth of *Candida*.

Candidal Paronychia

Candidal paronychia presents as edematous, erythematous nail folds with associated production of purulent discharge (Fig. 6-6). Prolonged immersion in water is a predisposing factor, and so bartenders, food handlers, and dishwashers are predisposed to develop this problem. Secondary infection of the paronychial area with bacteria such as *Staphylococcus aureus* can occur. It may be difficult to distinguish candidal from staphyloccoccal paronychia, and a Gram's stain and/or pottassium hydroxide preparation of the exudate may help.

Candidal Onychomycosis

There is some debate about whether *Candida* spp. are a significant pathogen in onychomycosis, but cultures of infected nails may reveal both dermatophyte and candidal organisms. *Candida* may be primarily pathogenic in a few select patients.

Systemic Candidiasis

Systemic candidiasis is a life-threatening infection that usually occurs in immunocompromised and debilitated patients. *Candida albicans* is the main pathogen iso-

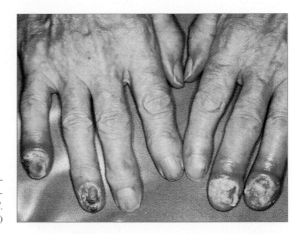

Figure 6-6

Chronic paronychia and onychia (nail infection). (From Freedberg I et al, eds: *Dermatology in General Medicine, 5th ed.* New York, McGraw-Hill, 1993, p. 2364.)

lated in systemic candidiasis, although *C. tropicalis* may be a cause, especially in leukemic patients. The single most important predisposing factor for the development of systemic disease is prolonged neutropenia. Hematogenous dissemination of *Candida* spp. may occur through a variety of mechanisms, including invasion through impaired epithelium or mucosa and an intravenous catheter. Clinical manifestations of systemic candidiasis include endophthalmitis, meningitis, esophagitis, endocarditis, hepatitis, myositis, nephritis, pneumonitis, osteomyelitis, and arthritis. The skin lesions of disseminated infections are variable but occur frequently as erythematous papules and pustules, especially on the extremities (Fig. 6-7). Cellulitis and abscesses are less common presentations of systemic disease.

Chronic Mucocutaneous Candidiasis

Chronic mucocutaneous candidiasis consists of a rare group of syndromes that are characterized by chronic candidal infection of the skin, nails, and mucous membranes in association with other features, such as autoimmune disease, endocrinopathy, and defects in cell-mediated immunity. Chronic mucocutaneous candidiasis usually presents by early childhood and is transmitted in an autosomal recessive, autosomal dominant, or sporadic pattern.

Evaluation

A scraping of a suspicious lesion prepared with 10 to 20% potassium hydroxide solution (KOH) is the first step in identifying a candidal infection. A positive KOH preparation yields multiple pseudohyphae when visualized under light microscopy (Fig. 6-8). False-negative tests may be seen when patients apply topical antifungal

Figure 6-7

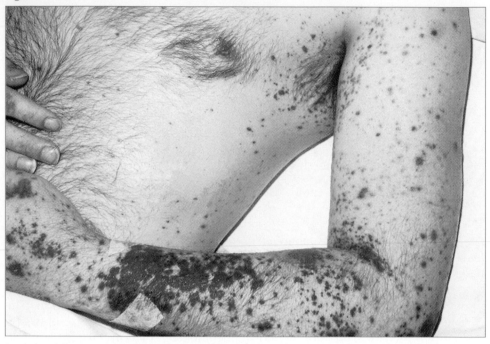

Septic candidiasis in an immunocompromised host.

agents that are available universally over the counter and by prescription. A skin biopsy is rarely needed for diagnosis but does demonstrate characteristic histopathologic findings. A fungal culture of mucocutaneous scrapings may aid in the identification of *Candida* spp., although this usually is necessary only in the setting of refractory disease and in immunocompromised hosts.

If systemic candidiasis is suspected, blood cultures obtained in the setting of disseminated disease are often negative. Clinical suspicion should guide treatment.

Treatment

Localized Treatment

OVERVIEW

When possible, factors that promote the development of *Candida* spp. should be eliminated. Treatment of the underlying systemic disease, such as diabetes mellitus, can aid immensely in the prevention of candidal colonization. Dentures should

Figure 6-8

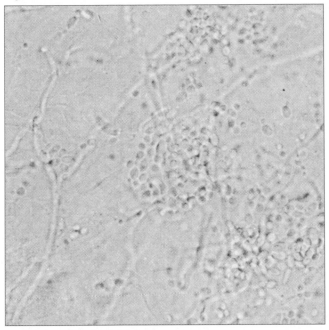

Candida in potassium hydroxide preparation. (From Freedberg I et al, eds: *Dermatology in General Medicine, 5th ed.* New York, McGraw-Hill, 1993, p. 2358.)

not be worn overnight and can be soaked in nystatin solution when they are not used. Dentures may be replaced by better-fitting appliances. Damp to dry soaks and drying agents such as zinc oxide paste, acetic acid (vinegar) solution, powders, and Burow's solution aid in eliminating excessive moisture in intertrigo patients. Frequent diaper changes and barrier creams help prevent diaper dermatitis.

TOPICAL   Topical antifungal preparations in the polyene (nystatin) or azole (clotrimazole, miconazole, econazole, ketoconazole, oxiconazole, sulconazole, butoconazole, and terconazole) class are the main treatments for cutaneous and mucosal candidiasis (Table 6-1). For patients with skin infections, we often suggest that the antifungal preparation be applied twice daily for 14 days. If the eruption does not clear in that time and the patient has been compliant, the physician should question the original diagnosis or treatment. Vaginal candidiasis responds to nightly intravaginal applications in regimens from 1 to 7 days. The newer allylamine class of antifungal medications (terbanfine and naftifine) has only moderate activity against *Candida* spp.; thus, these agents are expected to be less effective than are azole agents.

Nystatin works by binding yeast cell membrane ergosterol and promoting membrane leakage, and the azole medications work by inhibiting ergosterol synthesis.

Table 6-1

Selected Treatment Regimens for Candidiasis

TYPE	AGENT	REGIMEN
Cutaneous	Clotrimazole cream, lotion, or solution	Apply to skin bid for 2 weeks
	Fluconazole 100 mg	One tablet orally for 7 days
	Econazole cream	Apply to skin bid for 2 weeks
	Itraconazole 100 g	Two capsules orally for 3 to 7 days
	Ketoconazole cream	Apply to skin bid until healing complete
	Miconazole cream	Apply to skin bid for 2 weeks
	Nystatin cream	Apply to skin bid until healing complete
	Nystatin topical powder	Apply to skin bid until healing complete
	Oxiconazole cream or lotion	Apply to skin bid until healing complete
	Sulconazole cream or solution	Apply to skin bid for 2 weeks
Oral	Amphotericin B oral suspension	1 mL daily for 2 weeks
	Clotrimazole troche	One troche 5 times per day for 2 weeks
	Fluconazole 100 mg	Two tablets day 1 then one tablet orally for 13 days
	Nystatin pastilles	One to two pastilles 4 to 5 times per day for 2 weeks
Vulvovaginitis	Butoconazole cream	One applicator vaginally qhs for 3 days
		One applicator vaginally qhs for 1 day
	Clotrimazole vaginal cream	One applicator vaginally qhs for 7 days
	Clotrimazole 100 mg vaginal tablet	One tablet vaginally qhs for 7 days
		Two tablets vaginally for 3 days
	Fluconazole 150 mg	One tablet orally as a single dose
	Itraconazole 100 g	Two capsules orally for 3 days
	Miconazole vaginal cream	One applicator vaginally qhs for 7 days
	Miconazole vaginal suppository 100 mg	One suppository vaginally qhs for 7 days
	Miconazole vaginal suppository 200 mg	One suppository vaginally qhs for 3 days
	Nystatin 100,000 U vaginal tablet	One tablet vaginally qhs for 7 days
	Terconazole 0.4% vaginal cream	One applicator vaginally qhs for 7 days
	Terconazole 0.8% vaginal cream	One applicator vaginally qhs for 3 days
	Terconazole 80 mg vaginal suppository	One tablet vaginally qhs for 3 days
	Tioconazole vaginal ointment	One applicator vaginally as a single dose

Nystatin is available in suspension or pastille form and is helpful in treating candidal infections of the oral mucosa. Nystatin is also available as a powder and can be particularly effective in treating intertriginous candidiasis. It may be applied to the skin twice to four times daily.

Triamcinolone combined with nystatin also may have efficacy in patients with candidiasis with severe inflammation. Because of its potency, the corticosteroid triamcinolone should be used only for brief periods, such as one week.

The azole compounds are available in a wide variety of vehicles, including creams, lotions, solutions, and troches. Miconazole, clotrimazole, and terconazole, which are used mainly for treating vulvovaginal candidiasis, are available in creams and troches. A clotrimazole troche also may be useful for the treatment of oral or esophageal candidiasis. Most other azole compounds are used in the cream form for intertrigo, diaper dermatitis, and balanitis.

SYSTEMIC Oral agents can be used in conjunction with topical agents for resistant or recurrent candidiasis. Fluconazole is the most popular oral agent and has the greatest activity against *C. albicans*. It is useful for oropharyngeal candidiasis, especially in the HIV-positive population, and for vulvovaginal candidiasis. Vulvovaginal candidiasis often responds to a single 150-mg tablet. An alternative to treatment with this single dose is to use 100 mg daily for 1 week. Cutaneous candidiasis typically requires 1 to 2 weeks of fluconazole treatment. The side effects of fluconazole include drug interactions with cytochrome P450 enzyme-dependent medications (Table 6-2) and hepatitis.

Ketoconazole is an older oral agent with anticandidal activity. Because of the risk of severe hepatotoxicity, profound cytochrome P450 enzyme inhibition (see Table 6-2), and gynecomastia, this agent is rarely indicated.

Itraconazole is a triazole agent with an extraordinarily broad spectrum of activity against both yeasts and dermatophytes. It is clearly preferable to ketoconazole for infections because of its lower hepatotoxicity and less profound drug interactions. Itraconazole has been used successfully in patients with fluconazole-resistant disease. Nevertheless, like all azoles, it has drug interactions of note (see Table 6-2). Doses of 100 mg per day for 1 to 2 weeks are useful for most mucocutaneous candidal infections.

Amphotericin B is a polyene antifungal agent that is the mainstay of treatment for life-threatening *Candida* infections. Amphotericin B for this indication is administered intravenously. The side effects are significant and include fever, chills, hypotension, gastrointestinal upset, and impaired renal function. Renal function abnormalities may present as azotemia, renal tubular acidosis, or hypokalemia. For patients with disseminated candidiasis who are intolerant to amphotericin B, intravenous fluconazole is an option.

Table 6-2

Major Drug Interactions for Fluconazole, Ketoconazole, and Itraconazole

Antimicrobial agents	Erythromycin, clarithromycin, rifampin
Antihistaminic agents	Astemazole
Immunosuppressive agents	Tacrolimus, cyclosporine, methylprednisolone
Anticoagulant agents	Warfarin
Central nervous system agents	Phenytoin, midazolam, triazolam
Miscellaneous agents	Lovistatin, simvastatin, cimetidine, cisapride, Hypoglycemic agents (glyburide, glipizide, Tolbutamide, and others), theophylline, Zidovudine

Bibliography

Corrigan EM, Clancy RL, Dunkley ML, et al: Cellular immunity in recurrent vulvovaginal candidiasis. *Clin Exp Immunol* 111:574, 1998.

Del Rosso JQ, Zellis S, Gupta AK: Itraconazole in the treatment of superficial cutaneous and mucosal *Candida* infections. *J Am Osteopathal Assoc* 98:497, 1998.

Elliott KA: Managing patients with vulvovaginal candidiasis. *Nurse Pract* 23:44, 1998.

Fotos PG, Lilly JP: Clinical management of oral and perioral candidosis. *Dermatol Clin* 14:273, 1996.

Grossman ME, Silvers DN, Walther RR: Cutaneous manifestations of disseminated candidiasis. *J Am Acad Dermatol* 2:111, 1980.

Hay RJ: Antifungal therapy of yeast infections. *J Am Acad Dermatol* 31:S6, 1994.

Odds FC: Pathogenesis of candida infections. *J Am Acad Dermatol* 31:S2, 1994.

Ries AJ: Treatment of vaginal infections: Candidiasis, bacterial vaginosis, and trichomoniasis. *J Am Pharm Assoc* 37:563, 1997.

Schaaf VM, Perez-Stable EJ, Borchardt K: The limited value of symptoms and signs in the diagnosis of vaginal infections. *Arch Intern Med* 150:1929, 1990.

Sibbald RG, Landolt SJ, Toth D: Skin and diabetes. *Endocrinol Metabol Clin North Am* 25:463, 1996.

Sires UI, Mallory SB: Diaper dermatitis: How to treat and prevent. *Postgrad Med* 98:79, 1995.

Bacterial Folliculitis

Background   **Evaluation**
Etiology   **Treatment**
Clinical Presentation

Background

Folliculitis is a localized inflammatory process that originates in the hair follicle. It is a common dermatologic problem with multiple infectious and noninfectious causes. This chapter focuses on the most common type of folliculitis, which is due to bacteria. The most common pathogenic organism is *Staphylococcus aureus;* in certain circumstances, organisms such as *Pseudomonas aeruginosa* may be pathogenic.

Etiology

The initial element in the pathogenesis of folliculitis seems to be obstruction of the follicular orifice. This occlusion may be due to chemical occlusion, repetitive physical trauma, or abnormal production of keratinaceous material. Chemical occlusion with certain greases and oils, such as machine cutting oil, also may predispose a patient toward developing folliculitis. Repetitive physical trauma, as may be seen with friction from wearing tight clothing or epilation, may mechanically obstruct the hair follicle, leading to folliculitis. Keratosis pilaris, a condition in which there is abnormal production of keratinaceous material at the follicular orifice (on the extensor surface of the arms and thighs), may be associated with folliculitis. In many of these situations, cutaneous overhydration and maceration may lead to an increase in the number of bacteria on the skin. Organisms beneath the obstructed follicular ostium can then proliferate, leading to follicular inflammation.

Staphyloccal folliculitis is the major form of folliculitis, and chronic carriers of *S. aureus* are at high risk of developing this form. Some patients harbor *S. aureus* in relatively protected sites, such as the nose; these bacteria are not easily eradicated with antistaphyloccal antibiotic agents. Gram-negative folliculitis occurs most commonly in acne vulgaris patients who are receiving chronic oral antibiotic treatment. *Pseudomonas aeruginosa* folliculitis occurs most frequently in people who have spent time in whirlpools, hot tubs, or swimming pools that have been inadequately disinfected. Other unusual organisms have been reported in isolated cases. One of the more amusing examples is mud-wrestling-induced folliculitis caused by Enterobacteriaceae.

Clinical Presentation

Folliculitis presents as painless folliculocentric erythematous papules or pustules. Often the clinician can observe a tiny hair emanating from the center of several pustules (Fig 7-1). This form of folliculitis is most commonly found on the scalp, face, buttocks, and extremities. Involvement of the beard area is not uncommon (Fig. 7-2). Pustules arise in crops, and heal without scarring in 7 to 10 days. Widespread folliculitis may occur in some patients (Fig. 7-3).

Patients with gram-negative folliculitis usually provide a history of chronic antibiotic therapy for acne vulgaris or another chronic condition. A typical scenario is seen in a patient with acne disease that is difficult to control or acne that has flared recently despite appropriate systemic therapy. Gram-negative folliculitis has two distinct clinical presentations. The more prevalent form appears as multiple superficial pustules on the face and usually is caused by lactose-fermenting gram-negative bacilli. Less commonly, deep nodular cysts are present from which *Proteus* spp. may be cultured. The only way to distinguish this form of folliculitis from any other form is by means of bacterial culture.

Patients with *Pseudomonas* folliculitis often give a history of recent use of hot tubs or whirlpool baths. One to three days after infected water exposure, folliculitis develops explosively (Fig. 7-4). *Pseudomonas* folliculitis appears as multiple painful and/or pruritic folliculocentric erythematous papules and pustules. The lesions are scattered but tend to be most numerous in areas occluded by tight-fitting bathing

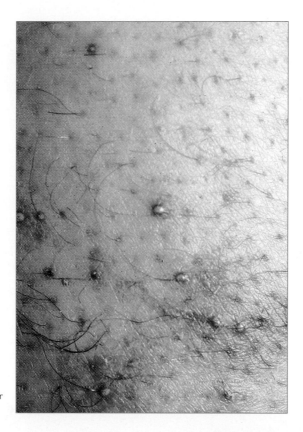

Figure 7-1

Pustules distributed at the orifices of hair follicles are characteristic of folliculitis.

suits. Individual lesions often resolve spontaneously within 2 weeks after the end of exposure.

Most commonly, all forms of bacterial folliculitis heal without scarring and complications. However, if the folliculitis extends more deeply or spreads to involve adjacent follicles, furuncles and carbuncles are formed. These lesions may require incision and drainage. Systemic infection is a rare complication that is seen mainly in immunocompromised hosts.

Evaluation

History and physical examination are usually suggestive of the diagnosis. In patients with an atypical presentation (e.g., there is so much excoriation that pustules cannot be identified) and those in whom conventional therapy is unsuccessful, clinicians should consider further evaluation, including a bacterial culture. A

Figure 7-2

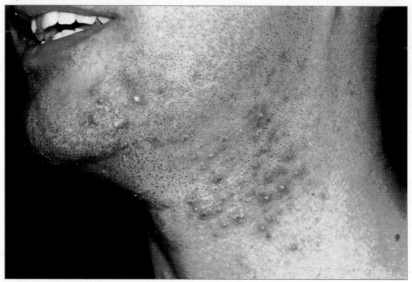

Folliculitis of the beard area. There are numerous pustules present in a follicular distribution. (From Fitzpatrick TB et al: *Color Atlas and Synopsis of Clinical Dermatology, 3/e*. New York, McGraw-Hill, 1995, p. 37.)

Figure 7-3

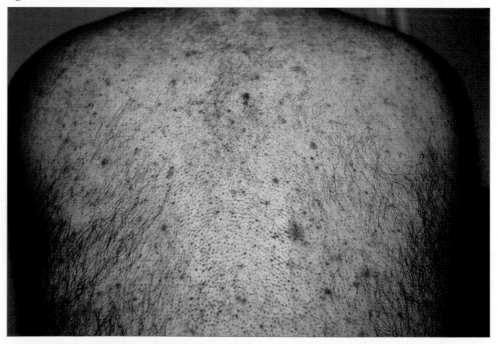

Widespread folliculitis commonly involves the trunk and extremities.

Figure 7-4

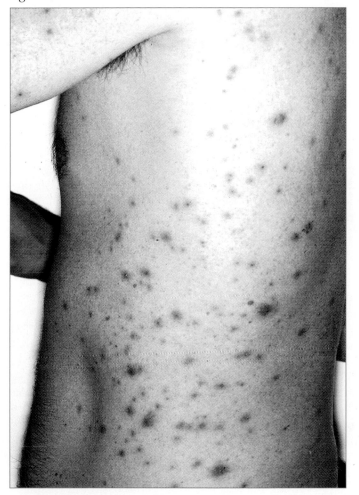

Hot tub folliculitis. Multiple follicular lesions (pustules and excoriations) appeared 3 days after the patient was in a hot tub. Because patients scratch pruritic folliculitis lesions, they may have many excoriations and few pustules. (From Fitzpatrick TB et al: *Color Atlas and Synopsis of Clinical Dermatology, 3/e.* New York, McGraw-Hill, 1995, p. 41.)

bacterial culture may reveal an organism that is sensitive to the antibiotic that has been prescribed, indicating poor adherence to the treatment regimen. Obtaining a punch or excisional biopsy specimen of a representative lesion may help exclude other types of folliculitis mimics, such as eosinophilic folliculitis (Ofuji's disease) (see Chap. 9).

Treatment

Staphylococcal folliculitis in a limited body area may be treated with twice-daily application of topical clindamycin solution (Cleocin) or erythromycin solution (T-Stat) or thrice-daily application of mupirocin ointment (Bactroban). Additionally, daily use of antibacterial soaps such as Dial and Lever 2000 may help reduce bacterial colonization. For recalcitrant or more extensive cases of folliculitis, oral antibiotic agents such as dicloxacillin, erythromycin, cephalexin, and amoxicillin with clavulanic acid (Augmentin) may be used. Patients with multiple recurrent cases are likely to be chronic nasal carriers of *S. aureus*. Eradication of the staphylococcal carrier state may be accomplished by means of intranasal application of mupirocin twice daily for 1 week each month. In general, mupirocin is well tolerated, but it may cause intranasal stinging. Alternatively, rifampin 300 mg twice daily for 1 month with the simultaneous use of an antistaphylococcal antibiotic agent such as cephalexin may clear the staphylococcal carrier state. Rifampin typically causes body fluids such as tears to change color, and this may stain contact lenses. Treatment with clindamycin 150 mg/d for 3 months has been found to be effective in eradicating the carrier state. Clindamycin has a significant risk of gastrointestinal toxicity (including pseudomembranous colitis), and clinicians should exercise caution in the use of this agent and probably reserve it as a second-line therapy for patients who have failed cephalexin or require clindamycin because of an oxicillin-resistant *S. aureus* infection. A few patients will have severe disease that is not responsive to this systemic therapy. Biopsy or culture may be needed to confirm the diagnosis and the susceptibility of the organism. Systemic isotretinoin may clear many types of folliculitis, presumably by changing the microenvironment of all the pilosebaceous units. Isotretinoin typically is used in doses of 1 mg/kg per day for 3 to 5 months. Despite the great efficacy of isotretinoin, therapy with this agent should be reserved for patients who have failed other approaches (see the published prescribing information and the discussion in Chapter 1). Clinicians should note that isotretinoin is extremely teratogenic, and pregnancy prevention is imperative.

Gram-negative folliculitis may be difficult to treat. The initial step in treatment should be to discontinue the use of the oral antibiotic that is being employed to treat the patient's acne. Subsequently, the patient should be started on appropriate oral antibiotics such as ampicillin, trimethoprim-sulfamethoxazole, and amoxicillin with clavulanic acid (Augmentin). While trimethoprim-sulfamethoxazole or amoxicillin with clavulanic acid may provide broader coverage, the added risks and expense of these agents may not be justified in most cases of folliculitis. Bacterial culture with antibiotic sensitivities is often helpful in guiding therapy. Treatment may have to be continued for months, with slow tapering of the antibiotic to prevent recurrences.

Isotretinoin has also been reported to be effective in treating gram-negative folliculitis. *Pseudomonas* folliculitis tends to resolve on its own in about 2 weeks and may not require treatment. Treatment with an antibiotic such as ciprofloxacin may shorten the duration. The most important aspect of treatment is to identify the source of the infection and then suggest that it be disinfected to prevent future infections.

Bibliography

Adler AI, Altman J: An outbreak of mud-wrestling-induced pustular dermatitis in college students: Dermatitis palaestrae limosae. *JAMA* 269:502, 1993.

Feingold DS: Staphylococcal and streptococcal pyodermas. *Semin Dermatol* 12:331, 1993.

Herman LE, Harawi SJ, Ghossein RA, et al: Folliculitis: A clinicopathologic review. *Pathol Ann* 26:201, 1991.

Hogan PA: *Pseudomonas* folliculitis. *Austral J Dermatol* 38:93, 1997.

Neubert U, Plewig G, Ruhfus A: Treatment of gram-negative folliculitis with isotretinoin. *Arch Dermatol Res* 278:307, 1986.

Noble WC: Gram-negative bacterial skin infections. *Semin Dermatol* 12:336, 1993.

Sadick NS: Current aspects of bacterial infections of the skin. *Dermatol Clin* 15:341, 1997.

Scott MJ Jr, Scott MJ III, Scott AM: Epilation. *Cutis* 46:216, 1990.

Herpes Simplex Virus Infections

Background

Herpes simplex virus (HSV) infection is one of the most commonly encountered human viral infections. HSV is a double-stranded DNA virus that is subdivided into two closely related types: HSV-1 and HSV-2. Oral-facial herpes is most commonly caused by HSV-1, while HSV-2 is most frequently implicated in genital lesions. It has been estimated that there are more than 500,000 new cases of genital HSV per year in the United States.

Etiology

Infection most often results from direct mucous membrane or skin contact between an infected individual and an uninfected individual. The risk factors for primary infection therefore include unprotected sexual contact and kissing. Other well-described but less commonly encountered modes of transmission include nonsexual rubbing, as occurs with wrestlers and rugby players, and herpetic whitlow, acquired when health or dental workers have contact with an infected patient.

Infections with either HSV-1 or HSV-2 occur either at mucosal surfaces or at sites of abraded skin. The virus infects epidermal and dermal cells, causing vesicles as a result of an influx of fluid containing free virus and degenerated epithelial cells. Sensory and autonomic nerve endings also are infected, with the virus traveling to the nucleus through retrograde axonal flow. In the sensory ganglia, the virus establishes latent infection for the lifetime of the host. During reactivation, the virus actively replicates, leading to lesions in the distribution of the affected nerve.

Once a patient has undergone primary infection, he or she may experience intermittent recurrences. Although they are not necessary for a recurrence to occur, certain factors put a patient at risk of a recurrence, including ultraviolet (UV) radiation, tissue injury, stress, and menstruation.

In recent years, it has been determined that asymptomatic virus shedding occurs with greater frequency than was previously recognized. Indeed, asymptomatic viral expression is much more common than are symptomatic episodes. Patients infected with HSV who have no signs or symptoms of active infection have cultures positive for virus between 1 and 7 percent of the days when they are tested. This asymptomatic shedding may result in infection of the sexual partners of an affected individual.

Clinical Presentation

For primary infection, patients may be able to give a history of exposure to an infected individual approximately 1 week before the onset of lesions. There also may be associated systemic complaints such as fever, malaise, myalgias, and regional adenopathy. Primary HSV infection may be asymptomatic or demonstrate lesions classically described as grouped umbilicated vesicles on an erythematous base. However, these lesions are not static. They may begin as erythematous papules or plaques and, after their vesicular phase, progress to pustules and then ulcerate over several days. Shallow "punched-out"-appearing ulcers may be all that is evident when the patient presents. If left untreated, the ulcers dry, crust, and heal over

2 to 3 weeks. Although the distribution of these lesions is most commonly perioral, labial, and genital, any cutaneous area may be affected. The most commonly seen primary infections with HSV are primary gingivostomatitis and primary genital herpes.

Primary Gingivostomatitis

Usually seen in children and young adults, this infection may range from mild to severe. Painful vesicles and ulcerations are noted on the tongue, buccal mucosa, hard and soft palate, lips, and face. In the mouth, the vesicles may coalesce to form plaques covered by a gray membrane (Fig. 8-1).

Primary Genital Herpes

Primary genital herpes usually presents with multiple erythematous vesicles that rupture and coalesce to form shallow "punched-out" exudative erosions (Figs. 8-2

Figure 8-1

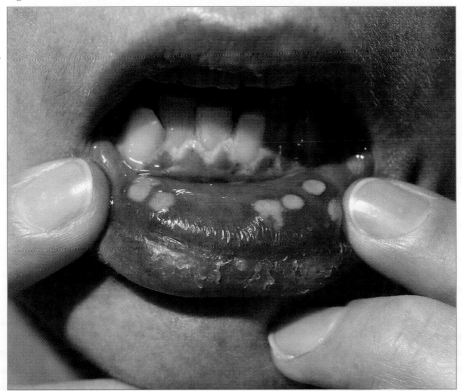

Primary herpetic gingivostomatitis. (From Fitzpatrick TB et al: *Color Atlas and Synopsis of Clinical Dermatology, 3/e.* New York, McGraw-Hill, 1995, p. 793.)

Figure 8-2

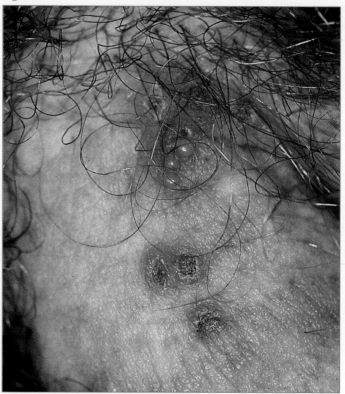

Penile herpes simplex. (From Freedberg I et al, eds: *Dermatology in General Medicine, 5/e.* New York, McGraw-Hill, 1999, p. 1370.)

and 8-3). Tender inguinal adenopathy may be noted. In women, cervical ulcers or cervicitis also may be present. Primary genital infection may be accompanied by clear mucoid discharge, severe dysuria, and even urinary retention.

With recurrent lesions, the patient may give a history of previous episodes of blisters or cold sores occurring in the exact same location (Fig. 8-4). The patient may describe a burning or tingling sensation a few hours before the eruption of the lesions. Recurrent lesions are usually less symptomatic than is the primary infection, with fewer lesions and faster healing. Recurrences are only rarely associated with systemic complaints.

Herpes infections may be impossible to differentiate from zoster infections. Herpes infections appear clinically identical to zoster infections, with dermatomal grouped umbilicated vesiculopustules on an erythematous base. As with zoster, the presenting symptoms may be mild to severe. Histologically, the two conditions are indistinguishable. Herpes has a tendency to be recurrent in the same dermatome. By contrast, zoster is rarely recurrent; when recurrent, it rarely is so in the same dermatome. Viral culture, immunoperoxidase staining of biopsy specimens, and polymerase chain reaction testing may help distinguish these conditions. Viral cul-

Figure 8-3

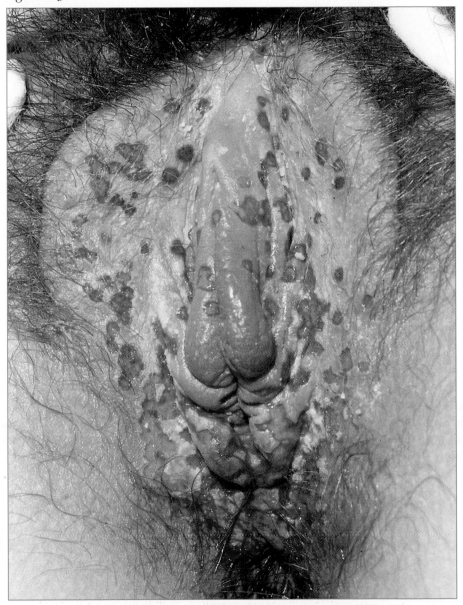

Herpetic vulvitis. (From Fitzpatrick TB et al: *Color Atlas and Synopsis of Clinical Dermatology, 3/e.* New York, McGraw-Hill, 1995, p. 911.)

ture is the least sensitive technique for detecting zoster infection, but it has reasonable sensitivity for simplex infections. Polymerase chain reaction testing is the most sensitive technique.

Herpes virus titers are relatively insensitive but are advocated by some clinicians.

Figure 8-4

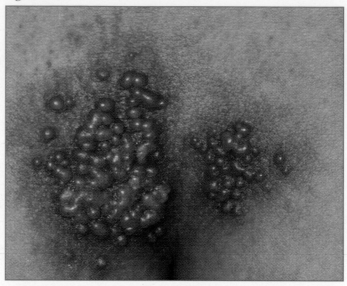

Recurrent lumbosacral herpes simplex. (From Freedberg I et al, eds: *Dermatology in General Medicine, 5/e.* New York, McGraw-Hill, 1999, p. 2420.)

Recurrent Oral-Facial Herpes

Also known as cold sores, the lesions of oral-facial herpes usually occur at the vermilion border of the lips (Fig. 8-5) or elsewhere on the face (Fig. 8-6) as an erythematous papule that rapidly evolves into a vesicle, and then a shallow ulceration.

Recurrent Genital Herpes

The severity and duration of symptoms are in recurrent genital herpes less than in the primary infection. A single or small cluster of typical lesions usually is noted. The recurrences usually start within the first year after primary infection and average three to four episodes per year.

Although these are the most commonly seen manifestations of HSV infection, other, less typical presentations also may be seen.

Neonatal Herpes

Neonatal herpes may present as characteristic herpetic lesions at days 4 to 7 of life or may involve the central nervous system (CNS) and visceral organs without cu-

Figure 8-5

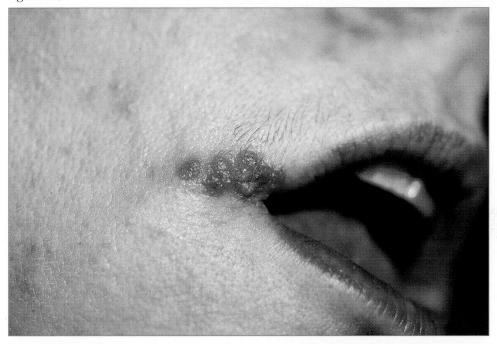

Herpes labialis: The cold sore.

taneous manifestations. Those at highest risk for neonatal herpes infection are persons whose mothers have acquired primary subclinical infection near term and are asymptomatically shedding virus.

Eczema Herpeticum

Eczema herpeticum may occur as widespread herpetic lesions in skin already compromised by processes such as atopic dermatitis, seborrheic dermatitis, and pemphigus, among other conditions (Fig. 8-7).

Herpetic Whitlow

This refers to primary or recurrent HSV infection of the fingers (Fig. 8-8) or hands (Fig. 8-9). It occurs most commonly in medical and dental personnel.

Herpes Gladiatorum

Cutaneous and ocular HSV-1 infections have been known to occur in wrestlers and rugby players, most frequently at the site of an abrasion or a break in the skin.

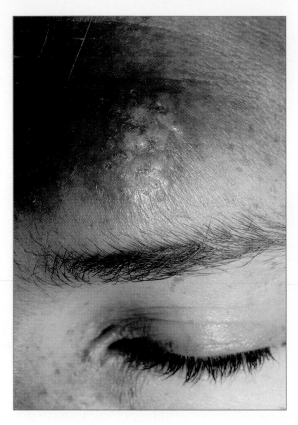

Figure 8-6

Facial herpes.

Immunocompromised Patients

The presentation is often atypical in immunocompromised patients, with more frequent recurrences, lesions persisting chronically as large ulcers, or even verrucous plaques. Also, atypical locations such as HSV esophagitis or proctitis may be seen.

In addition to the clinical situations described above, HSV infection may lead to other complications. Aseptic meningitis may be seen, most commonly in patients with primary genital herpes. Keratoconjunctivitis may occur when HSV involves the first division of the trigeminal nerve. Erythema multiforme may follow an eruption of recurrent herpes after 7 to 10 days. Additionally, genital ulcers caused by HSV infection may create an easy portal of entry for HIV infection. HSV-2 seropositivity, even in the absence of lesions, is an independent risk factor for HIV infection.

Figure 8-7

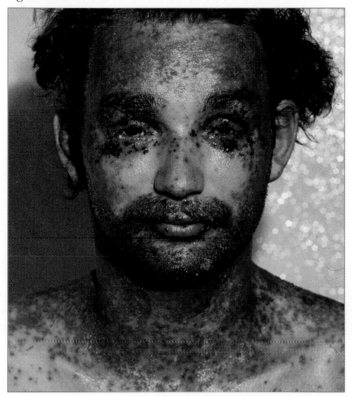

Eczema herpeticum. (From Freedberg I et al, eds: *Dermatology in General Medicine, 5/e.* New York, McGraw-Hill, 1999, p. 2421.)

Evaluation

The history of an acute onset of new or recurrent vesiculobullous lesions on an erythematous base is often highly suggestive of the diagnosis of HSV infection. However, adjunctive tests often are needed to confirm or establish the diagnosis. With any of the following techniques, the sensitivity of the test is highly dependent on the type of lesion sampled, with new vesicles giving the highest yield.

Tzanck smear may be performed rapidly in the office and should demonstrate viropathic multinucleated giant cells (Fig. 8-10). This technique requires a great deal of training, and methods of performing Tzanck smears are beyond the scope of this chapter. In brief, a sharp sterile blade is used to gently scrape cells from the bottom of an erosion or from the lower portion of a vesicle roof, and this material is smeared onto a microscope slide. A Wright's, Giemsa, Diff-Quik, or

Figure 8-8

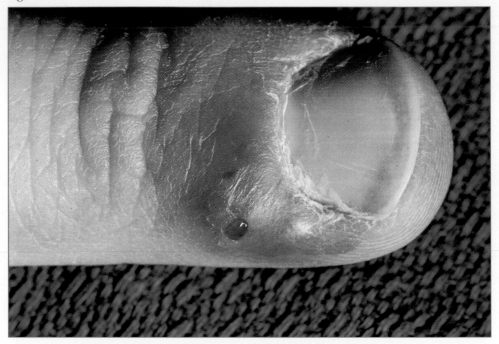

Herpetic whitlow of the finger.

similar staining technique allows one to see the viropathic cells. This technique does not differentiate HSV from varicella zoster virus.

Viral culture should grow HSV within 48 h. It is capable of differentiating HSV-1, HSV-2, and varicella zostervirus (VZV). As in the Tzanck procedure, a sharp sterile blade is used to gently scrape cells from the bottom of an erosion or from the lower portion of a vesicle roof, and this material is placed into a viral transport medium. Immediate transportation to a viral laboratory improves diagnostic sensitivity.

Skin biopsy specimen examination may be suggestive of HSV and may be useful in ruling out other suspected conditions. Unfortunately, the several-day period required to receive histopathologic results often precludes an acute diagnosis. HSV and zoster have identical microscopic features. Accordingly, skin biopsy is rarely performed except when the clinical morphology is bizarre.

In certain institutions, polymerase chain reaction (PCR) may also be used to detect HSV DNA. This is the fastest, most reliable, and most sensitive technique. In contrast to viral culture, PCR is less subject to specimen degradation, which quickly occurs if specimens are not immediately inoculated into culture media. Accordingly, the PCR technique is rapidly becoming the criterion standard for diagnosis and may replace all other techniques except Tzanck examination.

Figure 8-9

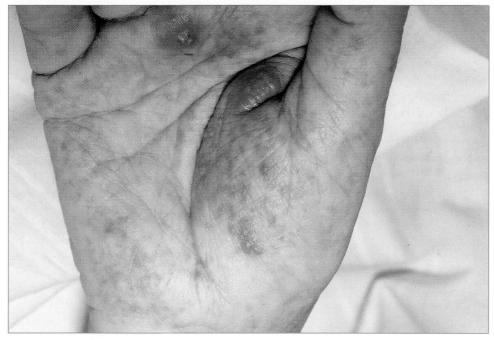

Herpes simplex virus of the hand.

Treatment

Overview

Patient education is an important first step in the management of patients with HSV infection. Particularly for genital HSV infection, counseling should be given regarding the natural history of herpes, sexual and perinatal transmission, and methods to reduce such transmission. Patients should be informed that the lesions may recur, usually in the same location. They should be instructed that lesional contact should be avoided from prodrome until complete re-epithelialization. Since asymptomatic shedding of intact viral particles commonly occurs, this topic should be addressed clearly with patients. Additionally, condom use to prevent the transmission of genital HSV infection is prudent, even between clinical recurrences, because of the possibility of asymptomatic shedding of the virus. Orolabial HSV frequently is triggered by intense sun exposure, and patients should use sunscreen on the face and lip balm containing a sunscreen.

Treatment of herpetic infections is suppressive, not curative. Systemic treatment is clearly much more effective than is topical treatment. However, if systemic treatment is contraindicated or refused, topical treatment may play a minor role in viral suppression.

Systemic Therapy

TREATMENT OF ACUTE INFECTION

For patients with primary HSV infection, whether orofacial or genital, the best studied treatment is acyclovir 200 mg five times daily for 7 to 10 days. This treatment has been shown to decrease pain, new lesion formation, the duration of viral shedding, and the time to crusting and resolution. Since acyclovir is poorly absorbed and requires administration five times per day, it is no longer a treatment of choice.

Treatment options that are superior to acyclovir include famciclovir 250 mg three times daily for 7 to 10 days and valacyclivir 500 mg orally twice a day for 7 to 10 days. Famciclovir and valacyclovir are better absorbed than is acyclovir and probably are more effective because of the need for less frequent dosing. The only patient groups for which acyclovir remains appropriate are children, as there is no other antiherpetic antivarial elixir, and immunocompromised hosts, in whom the use of valacyclovir and famciclovir has not been studied adequately. Valacyclovir should be used with extreme caution in immunocompromised patients because of

Figure 8-10

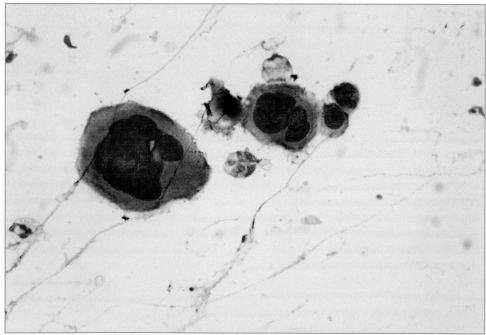

Grouped vesiculopustules on an erythematous base, characteristic of herpes simplex.

occurrences of thrombotic thrombocytopenic purpura in some patients during clinical trials. None of these treatments has been found to decrease the chance of future recurrences.

TREATMENT OF RECURRENT DISEASE

In treating recurrences of HSV infection, acyclovir, famciclovir, and valacyclovir have all been found to be effective. Regardless of which one is used, these medications are more effective the earlier they are started. We recommend having patients get the prescription filled for the medication and keep it at home. They are instructed to begin taking the medication at the first tingling or other prodromal symptom they notice. Treatment regimens for recurrent HSV episodes for the various antiviral agents include the following:

Acyclovir 200 mg five times a day for 5 days
Acyclovir 400 mg three times a day for 5 days
Famciclovir 125 mg twice daily for 5 days
Valacyclovir 500 mg twice daily for 5 days

In certain situations, one may wish to treat the patient prophylactically with antiviral therapy to prevent recurrences. Patients who are scheduled to undergo major cosmetic surgery on the face or extensive dental work should receive antiviral therapy in the doses used for recurrent HSV infections. Treatment should begin 2 days before the surgical procedure and continue for 5 days afterward.

Suppressive therapy should be considered in patients who develop frequent recurrences and patients who develop erythema multiforme after HSV recurrences. Patients may be started on chronic therapy with either acyclovir 400 mg twice daily or valacyclovir 1 g once daily or famciclovir 250 mg twice daily. Once adequate suppression has been established, patients should be tapered to the minimal effective dose.

Topical Therapy

Topical antiviral agents such as penciclovir (Denavir) have been found to decrease the duration of outbreaks slightly. In patients who refuse more effective systemic therapy and patients who believe that topical therapy is effective, these agents may be prescribed safely. Denavir is a cream that should be applied every two waking hours for 4 days. It is unknown whether topical antiviral treatment can augment the efficacy of systemic agents.

Bibliography

Erlich KS: Management of herpes simplex and varicella-zoster virus infections. *West J Med* 166:211, 1997.
Gulick R, in Arndt KA et al (eds): *Cutaneous Medicine and Surgery*. Philadelphia, Saunders, 1996, pp. 1074–1078.
Pereira FA: Herpes simplex: Evolving concepts. *J Am Acad Dermatol* 35:503, 1996.

Rubben A, Baron JM, Grussendorf-Conen EI: Routine detection of herpes simplex virus and varicella zoster virus by polymerase chain reaction reveals that initial herpes zoster is frequently misdiagnosed as herpes simplex. *Br J Dermatol* 137:259, 1997.

Zirn JR, Tompkins SD, Huie C, Shea CR: Rapid detection and distinction of cutaneous herpesvirus infections by direct immunofluorescence. *J Am Acad Dermatol* 33:724, 1995.

Chapter 9

Human Immunodeficiency Virus and Skin Disease

Background
Risk Factors
Pathophysiology
Symptoms
Physical Examination
- General Notes
- Infection
- Neoplasia
- Inflammatory Disorders

Evaluation
- Infection
- Neoplasm
- Inflammatory Disorders

Management and Treatment
- Infection
- Neoplastic Disease
- Inflammatory Disorders

Background

The prevalence of skin disease is quite high in patients with advanced Human Immunodeficiency Virus (HIV) infections. The primary infection with HIV may be associated with an infectious exanthem (Fig. 9-1). Other skin manifestations include infections, inflammatory disorders, malignancies, and miscellaneous conditions. Some of these cutaneous manifestations, such as disseminated skin lesions of histoplasmosis or cyrptococcosis, or Kaposi's sarcoma may be AIDS-defining. They also may be disfiguring and disabling. It is worth remembering that patients with advanced HIV disease are subject to getting the same diseases that all other people are subject to getting, but many diseases present more commonly in the immunocompromised host. Essentially all of the conditions mentioned in this chapter also occur in other immunocompromised hosts, including patients with cancer and those on immunosuppressive medications.

Figure 9-1

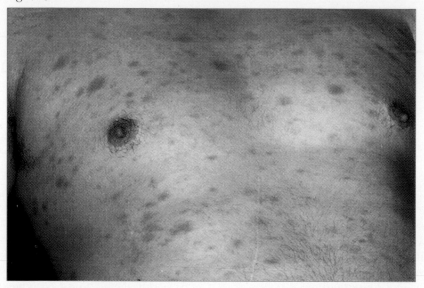

Eruption associated with primary infection with HIV. This eruption of multiple erythematous macules and papules is similar to drug eruption and to other viral exanthems.

Risk Factors

The occurrence and severity of HIV-associated dermatoses may be influenced by the patient's CD4+ count, with lower counts contributing to a greater risk of skin disease. Many of the skin findings in HIV disease are found in more advanced or end stages. Kaposi's sarcoma is found most commonly in homosexual men.

Pathophysiology

Many of the infectious manifestations of HIV-associated skin disorders relate to impaired cell-mediated immunity, leading to extensive or recalcitrant viral or fungal infections. In addition, there is an increased incidence of bacterial infections in HIV-positive patients, suggesting an impairment in humoral immunity. Neoplasms may arise in this patient population as a result of the opportunistic oncogenic infections that occur in advanced HIV disease.

Kaposi's sarcoma is felt to result from concurrent infection with human herpes virus 8 (HHV-8). This virus exists in normal adults but is more commonly expressed in an immunocompromised host.

Symptoms

HIV infection may exacerbate preexisting dermatoses or predispose a patient to develop opportunistic infections. As the degree of immunosuppression becomes more severe, dermatoses often become more extensive and resistant to treatment. Many skin disorders associated with HIV disease, such as molluscum contagiosum and Kaposi's sarcoma, can be physically disfiguring. Other problems, such as oral candidiasis and aphthae, may be so painful that the ability to eat is compromised. Of course, the specific symptom complex depends on the nature of the condition.

Physical Examination

General Notes

In immunodeficient individuals, the clinical appearance of lesions may be atypical. Accordingly, the clinician should consider a lower threshold for biopsy and culture than he or she would in immunocompetent individuals.

Infection

Staphylococcus aureus infections can be primary, or the bacteria may secondarily infect preexisting dermatoses. The primary staphylococcal infections include folliculitis, which manifests as multiple follicular-based erythematous papules and pustules in areas such as the buttocks, chest, back, and thighs. Impetigo presents as honey-colored crusted plaques and may include flaccid bullous lesions that are commonly found in the axilla or groin area. Furuncles and carbuncles are erythematous subcutaneous tender nodules that may have associated draining pus. Cellulitis may be due to either staphylococcal or streptococcal organisms.

Bacillary angiomatosis is caused by the organism *Bartonella henselae*. These vascular lesions are characterized by reddish purple papules, nodules, and from one to multiple plaques and are found anywhere on the cutaneous surface (Fig. 9-2). Care should be taken to not confuse Kaposi's sarcoma with bacillary angiomatosis.

Figure 9-2

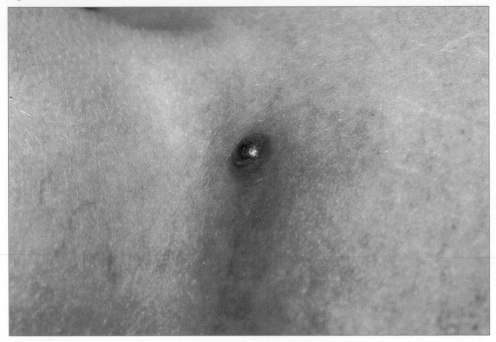

Bacillary angiomatosis. This lesion of bacillary angiomatosis appears similar to pyogenic granuloma or Kaposi sarcoma.

Syphilis is manifested in HIV-positive patients in the same way it is manifested in HIV-negative patients. The primary disease presents as a firm, nontender rubbery ulcer, usually in the genital area. Secondary syphilis has a wide variety of configurations, including papular or macular lesions (Fig. 9-3), especially with papulosquamous lesions of the palms and soles. Syphilis may progress more rapidly in immunocompromised hosts, and neurologic disease may occur more quickly than it does in a nonimmunocompromised host.

Dermatophytosis in patients who are positive for the AIDS virus has a presentation similar to that of dermatophyte infections in non-HIV-infected patients. It has a tendency to present in a more widespread fashion. Onychomycosis, or nail fungal infection, may present with either the common distal subungual onychomycosis pattern or as proximal subungual onycholysis.

Candidiasis, when it involves the vulvar or vaginal area, presents as erythematous plaques that may have an associated white exudate, satellite pustules, or the presence of cheesy vaginal discharge. The oropharynx is the most common site of mucosal candidiasis, and involvement may extend into the esophagus or trachea. The most common presentation of oropharyngeal candidiasis is white plaques that may bleed upon scraping with a tongue blade and are commonly found on the buccal mucosa, the soft palate, and the dorsum of the tongue. An erythematous or hyperplastic variety also exists.

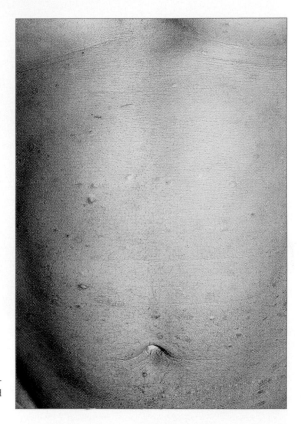

Figure 9-3

An AIDS patient presenting with a widespread papular eruption and who proved to have secondary syphilis.

Pityrosporum spp. cause tinea versicolor, which presents as multiple white scaling oval patches involving the neck, back, and chest. *Pityrosporum* folliculitis is characterized by multiple erythematous follicular-based papules on the trunk.

Deep fungal and mycobacterial infections are more common in an immunocompromised host. Infections with histoplasmosis, coccidioidomycosis, blastomycosis, and mycobacteria other than *Mycobacterium tuberculosis* may present as erythematous to ulcerating macules, papules, plaques, or tumors (Figs. 9-4 and 9-5).

Primary varicella infection usually occurs in childhood. If it presents later in an HIV-positive patient, the infection may be much more severe.

Herpes simplex and herpes zoster present as multiple grouped vesicles that quickly progress to ulcerations. These lesions are found primarily in the oral and genital areas in cases of herpes simplex virus (HSV) (Fig. 9-6) and in a dermatomal distribution in cases of herpes zoster (Fig. 9-7). Both HSV and zoster may present in acute or chronic forms and may display a dermatomal distribution. Large perianal and perioral ulcers may occur with HSV and are difficult to differentiate clinically from similar ulcers caused by cytomegalovirus. Unlike in nonimmunocompromised hosts, zoster may be recurrent in this population. Chronic nonhealing forms of zoster and herpes simplex may occur.

Figure 9-4

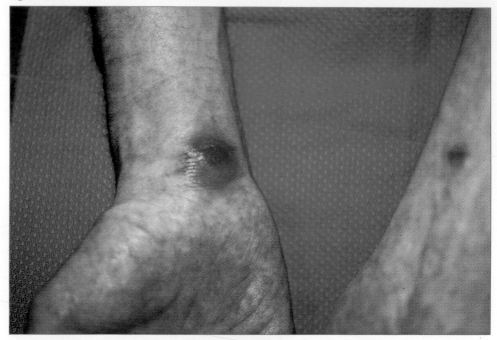

Rapidly enlarging erythematous nodules that grew *Mycobacterium haemophilum* in culture.

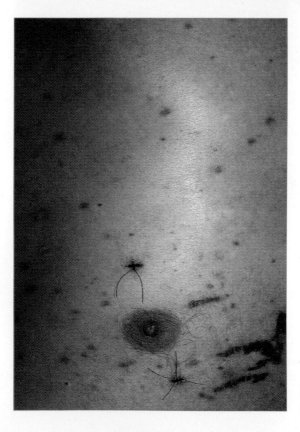

Figure 9-5

Multiple widespread erythematous papules that proved to be disseminated *cryptococcosus*.

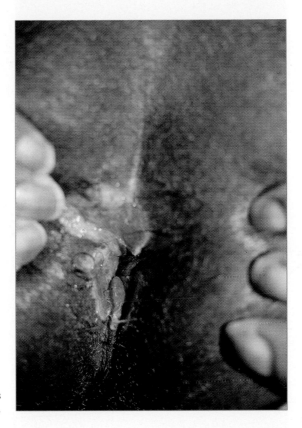

Figure 9-6

Chronic anogenital herpes simplex virus infection resistant to acyclovir therapy.

Molluscum contagiosum results from infection with a poxvirus and often presents as multiple pearly, umbilicated papules, especially on the face and genital area (Figs. 9-8 and 9-9). The papules may reach sizes exceeding 1 cm in HIV-positive patients.

Human papillomavirus infection is common in the HIV-positive population. These warts do not differ in clinical appearance from warts on patients who are not infected with HIV. However, some of the largest warts seen by the authors have been in patients with advanced HIV disease. Different wart varieties exist, including verrucous hyperkeratotic papules (common warts), flesh-colored flat-topped papules (flat warts), and hyperkeratotic plaques on the bottom of the feet (plantar warts). Genital warts, which range in morphology from isolated flesh-colored papules to pedunculated "cauliflower-like" masses, are also common in patients with HIV infection.

Epstein-Barr virus may cause oral hairy leukoplakia, which presents as shaggy white plaques on the lateral aspect of the tongue.

Scabies may be present with erythematous macules and papules in the web spaces, gluteal cleft, and genitalia. More commonly, the appearance is that of crusted (Norwegian) scabies with hyperkeratotic patches and plaques in a generalized distribution. The hyperkeratotic debris under fingernails teems with mites.

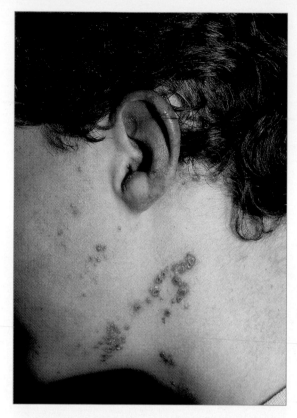

Figure 9-7

Zoster presenting in a young AIDS patient in a dermatomal distribution.

Figure 9-8

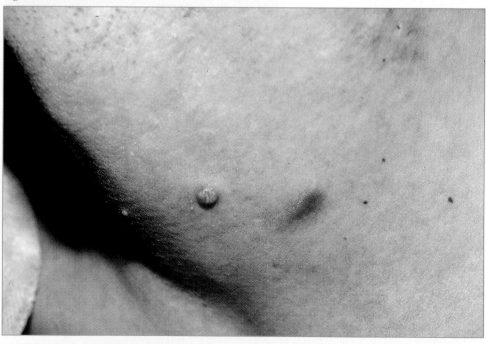

A molluscum lesion on the neck of an AIDS patient, approximately 2 cm from a Kaposi's sarcoma lesion.

Figure 9-9

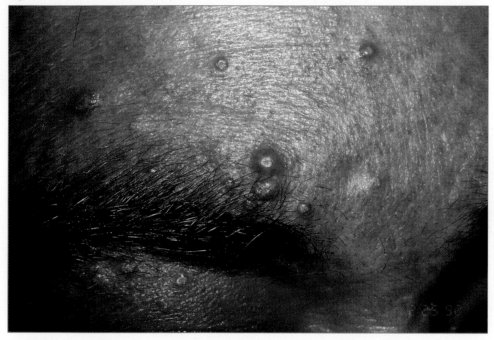

Molluscum contagiosum. The multiple small dome-shaped umbilicated papules are typical of molluscum contagiosum.

Neoplasia

Kaposi's sarcoma usually begins as erythematous macules or papules and develops into violaceous plaques and nodules that are usually oval in shape (Figs. 9-10 and 9-11). These lesions are found on the trunk, leg, arm, face, and oral cavity and usually lack symmetry. On the trunk, multiple lesions can present in a "Christmas tree" pattern. Although Kaposi's sarcoma may be found in nonimmunocompromised hosts, it can be AIDS-defining.

Inflammatory Disorders

Seborrheic dermatitis is characterized by erythematous scaling waxy plaques in the scalp, ears, eyebrows, and nasolabial folds. Occasionally there is also involvement on the chest, axilla, and pubic area. This dermatosis can be quite severe in patients with HIV infection. Although listed as an inflammatory rather than an infectious disorder, seborrheic dermatitis may be related to overgrowth of *Pityrosporum* yeast species or to an abnormal host response to this commensal organism.

Psoriasis is characterized by well-circumscribed erythematous plaques with thick, silvery scaling. The distribution usually includes the elbows, knees, and trunk but

Figure 9-10

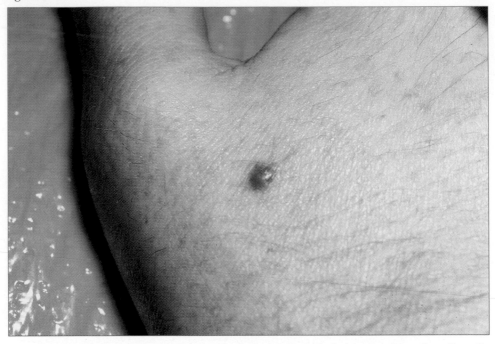

A nondescript erythematous papule that was shown by histopathologic interpretation to be a Kaposi's sarcoma.

may be extensive and generalized. There may be an associated nail dystrophy with hyperkeratosis, distal onycholysis, and pitting as well as arthritis.

Atopic dermatitis associated with HIV disease appears identical to atopic dermatitis in patients not infected with HIV. However, it may be more severe and extensive. Atopic dermatitis is characterized by scaling, patchy erythematous plaques involving the face and neck, areas of the trunk, antecubital fossae, hands, and feet.

Drug eruptions usually present as a morbilliform, generalized erythematous eruption involving primarily the trunk and proximal extremities. These eruptions tend to be more common in HIV-positive patients. Other forms of drug eruptions, including fixed drug eruption, which presents as a hyperpigmented circular plaque, and Stevens-Johnson syndrome, which is characterized by generalized erythroderma with bullae and crusted plaques involving the conjunctiva and oral and genital mucous membranes, also occur more frequently in HIV-positive patients.

Eosinophilic folliculitis is characterized by monomorphous erythematous papules and pustules found primarily on the face and trunk in HIV-positive individuals. This intensely pruritic condition may present only as excoriated papules.

Pruritic papular eruption is characterized by intensely itchy papules in a localized or, more commonly, generalized distribution. Skin-colored papules and nodules may develop into chronic lesions that are excoriated and hyperpigmented.

Figure 9-11

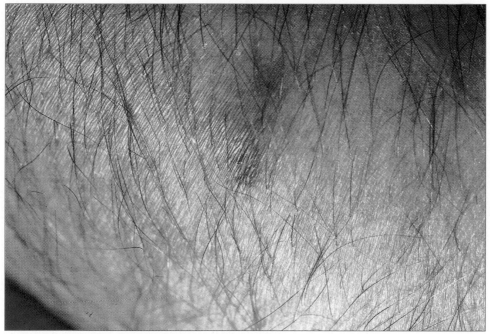

Kaposi's sarcoma. The ill-defined and asymmetric appearance of this vascular lesion is a worrisome sign.

Oral aphthae present as multiple shallow erosions from 1 mm to 1 cm in diameter on the oral mucosa. They may extend into the pharynx and esophagus and may cause severe pain and dysphagia.

Acquired ichthyosis is characterized by exceptionally dry, cracked skin. The lesions are seen most commonly on the extremities but can be generalized.

Evaluation

Infection

The evaluation of any lesion suspicious for infection in an HIV-positive patient may include culture for bacteria, fungus, or virus or a skin biopsy. The clinician should be aware that common infections may present in unusual ways and that uncommon infections may present at any time. Some diagnoses may be made exclusively on clinical grounds. The lesions of folliculitis may be cultured for staphylococcal organisms or require a potassium hydroxide (KOH) preparation to exclude *Pity-rosporum* organisms. Alternatively, a skin biopsy may be required. Any lesion suspicious for a manifestation of syphilis should have appropriate dark-field examination performed if possible and have serologic testing performed initially and afterward to follow titers. A KOH examination with or without a confirmatory fungal culture should be considered for dermatophytosis or candidiasis. When this procedure is done, hyphae and spores are seen with fungal processes and pseudohyphae are seen with candidal processes. Other fungal and mycobacterial infections require specific culture media.

Any ulcerative lesion, especially in the perioral or perianal area, should be evaluated by means of a Tzanck preparation to identify viropathic multinucleated giant cells. A viral culture or another diagnostic technique (e.g., polymerase chain reaction) should be done on these ulcers to identify herpes simplex or cytomegalovirus (CMV). Occasionally, pathognomonic findings of herpetic infections or CMV may be seen on a skin biopsy done at the ulcer edge. Molluscum contagiosum usually is identified by its characteristic clinical appearance, but other infections, such as disseminated cryptococcus, may produce lesions with a similar appearance. When the diagnosis is in doubt, consider obtaining a punch or shave biopsy of the lesion. White plaques in the oral cavity usually can be differentiated as *Candida* versus oral hairy leukoplakia by the clinical appearance and microscopic examination of a wet preparation. However, overlap in clinical features may force the clinician to obtain a biopsy specimen.

Neoplasm

The diagnosis of all vascular lesions should be confirmed with a punch or shave biopsy. Kaposi's sarcoma cannot be differentiated clinically from bacillary angiomatosis. By contrast, the characteristic changes of Kaposi's sarcoma or bacillary angiomatosis are found on histopathologic samples. Cutaneous lymphomas may be present and are best diagnosed by means of skin biopsy specimen interpretation.

Inflammatory Disorders

The diagnosis of inflammatory disorders is often made exclusively on clinical grounds. A very severe or atypical presentation of a common skin disease such as seborrheic dermatitis may alert the physician to the presence of HIV infection. A skin biopsy may be helpful in establishing the diagnosis if there is a question about the etiology of an eruption.

Management and Treatment

Infection

Staphylococcus aureus may respond to a course of a penicillinase-resistant penicillin, a cephalosporin, or erythromycin. Extensive or deep-seated infection may require a concurrent antibiotic such as rifampin 300 mg twice daily for 7 to 30 days. Recurrent infections may benefit from prophylactic topical or oral antibiotics as well as mupirocin ointment applied in the nares to decrease staphylococcal carriage.

Bacillary angiomatosis may respond to systemic treatment with erythromycin 1 to 2 g per day for 2 to 3 months. Rifampin also has been shown to be effective.

Syphilis should be treated in compliance with the recommendations of the Centers for Disease Control and Prevention (CDC). The CDC recommends intramuscular injection of benzathine G penicillin 2.4 million units for the treatment of primary and secondary syphilis in HIV-infected patients; this is the same as the treatment for patients who are HIV-negative. The patient must undergo cerebrospinal fluid (CSF) examination and be followed closely for evidence of treatment failure. Some experts recommend three weekly treatments with benzathine G penicillin 2.4 million units intramuscularly or the addition of other antibiotics to penicillin. A patient with latent syphilis and a negative CSF examination should be treated with a weekly intramuscular injection of benzathine G penicillin 2.4 million units for 3 weeks.

Dermatophytosis, when limited to a few localized sites, may respond well to topical azole antifungal agents (e.g., sulconazole, econazole, oxiconazole) or allyl amine antifungal agents (e.g., terbinafine or naftifine). When applied twice daily for 3 to 4 weeks, this is usually curative. Tinea unguium or extensive tinea infections may require a course of an oral antifungal agent such as terbinafine.

Candida paronychia usually is treated adequately with a twice-daily application of topical azole (e.g., sulconazole, econazole, oxiconazole) antifungal agents. Cutaneous infections also often respond to this regimen. Oral or esophageal candidiasis may respond to therapy with clotrimazole troches. Resistant or extensive cutaneous oral candidiasis may require a course of oral antifungal agents such as itraconazole and fluconazole. Nail candidal infections may require months of itraconazole or fluconazole to eradicate the infection.

Pityrosporum folliculitis requires either topical or oral azole antifungal agents. Pityriasis (tinea) versicolor usually responds to a combination of a single dose of ketoconazole or itraconazole 400 mg followed by topical overnight application of selenium sulfide 2.5% lotion weekly for 1 month.

Primary varicella infections should be treated aggressively with acyclovir until clearance is observed. Much longer treatment durations may be required.

Herpes simplex or zoster should be treated with a 5- to 7-day course of an oral antiviral agent such as acyclovir 800 mg five times per day. Since it is often unclear whether the presenting eruption is herpes simplex or zoster, higher doses are recommended for uncomplicated cases of herpes simplex or zoster. The use of newer antiviral agents such as valacyclovir and famciclovir has not been established in this population. Disseminated herpes simplex or zoster infections as well as severe ulcerative cases of HSV require intravenous acyclovir. An acyclovir-resistant strain of HSV exists and may require treatment with famciclovir or foscarnet.

Molluscum contagiosum may be amenable to destructive methods such as cryosurgery and light electrodesiccation. These lesions are notorious for their recurrence.

Human papillomavirus infections may be treated with topical agents or ablative techniques, as described in Chap. 13.

Topical therapies such as tretinoin and podophyllin have been effective for treatment of Epstein-Barr virus infection. Systemic acyclovir or zidovudine and surgical excision have been described as successful treatments.

Scabies therapy should be more thorough than it is in nonimmunocompromised patients, since HIV patients are more likely to host numerous mites. Therefore, a single application of permethrin (5%) cream or lindane is not likely to succeed. Although precise guidelines are unavailable for this condition, clinicians should consider treating severely affected immunocompromised hosts with at least four topical treatments over 2 weeks. Care should be taken to treat all contacts of the index patient and follow the patient to therapeutic response.

Neoplastic Disease

Kaposi's sarcoma treatment is important to reduce pain and disfigurement. Local destructive therapy such as liquid nitrogen cryotherapy can be used to treat individual lesions. Intralesional injection of chemotherapeutic agents such as vinblastine as well as radiation therapy are alternative treatments. Extensive, life-threatening internal involvement requires systemic chemotherapy. With all forms of therapy, recurrences are common.

Inflammatory Disorders

Seborrheic dermatitis may respond to a combination of topical corticosteroid agents such as hydrocortisone and antifungal creams or shampoos containing ketoconazole, selenium sulfide, or pyrithione zinc. Treatment ameliorates the condition but is not curative. Severe involvement may require midpotency topical corticosteroid agents such as fluticasone, triamcinolone, and hydrocortisone valerate in areas such as the face, where they generally are not applied for limited periods.

Psoriasis treatment differs slightly from psoriasis treatment in nonimmunocompromised hosts (see Chap. 3). Systemic immunosuppressive agents such as cyclosporine and methotrexate generally are not used in the setting of HIV disease.

Oral retinoid agents such as acitretin are systemic alternatives that do not affect the patient's immune status.

Atopic dermatitis is treated similarly to the way it is treated in nonimmuno-compromised patients, using topical corticosteroid and anesthetic agents. Antibiotic therapy may be used for secondary infections.

Drug eruptions are best approached by attempting to identify the probable causative agent or agents and discontinuing them. Treatment is aimed at alleviating symptoms and consists of topical corticosteroids and other antipruritic agents. More severe drug eruptions, such as Stevens-Johnson syndrome and toxic epidermal necrolysis, usually require hospitalization.

Eosinophilic folliculitis is notoriously difficult to manage. Empirical treatment with topical corticosteroid agents, dapsone, antimicrobial therapy, isotretinoin, or ultraviolet B (UVB) phototherapy may be helpful. The disease course is often chronic and persistent.

Pruritic papular eruption typically waxes and wanes and is generally resistant to oral antihistamine and topical steroid therapy. UVB and psorafen with ultraviolet A (PUVA) phototherapy have been successful in many patients and are considered safe.

Oral aphthae may improve with the use of ultrapotent topical corticosteroid agents applied four times per day to the individual lesions. Systemic corticosteroids may be helpful but generally are avoided in this population. Systemic thalidomide treatment is rapidly effective and is the treatment of choice for severe or extensive involvement. Thalidomide is highly teratogenic, and accordingly, fetal exposure prevention is essential. Thalidomide also may be neurotoxic in patients, and careful monitoring for this peripheral neuropathy is strongly recommended.

Aquired ichthyosis may respond to topical emollients applied twice daily and may require the addition of an alphahydroxy acid such as ammonium lactate cream twice daily.

Bibliography

Bason MM, Berger TG, Nesbitt LT Jr: Pruritic papular eruption of HIV-disease. *Int J Dermatol* 32:784, 1993.

Buchness MR, Lim HW, Hatcher VA, et al: Ultraviolet B phototherapy of eosinophilic pustular follicultits in patients with the acquired immunodeficiency syndrome. *New Engl J Med* 318:1183, 1988.

Buchness MR, Sanchez M: HIV-associated pruritus. *Clin Dermatol* 9:111, 1991.

Goldman GD, Bolognia JL: HIV-related skin disease: Inflammatory dermatoses. *J Respir Dis* 17:914, 1996.

Hoover WD Jr, Lang PG: Pruritus in HIV infection. *J Am Acad Dermatol* 24:1020, 1991.

Ishii N, Nishiyama T, Sugita Y, et al: Pruritic papular eruption of the acquired immunodeficiency syndrome. *Acta Dermatol Venereol* 74:219, 1994.

Jewell ME, Sweet DE: Oral and dermatologic manifestations of HIV infection. *Postgrad Med* 96:105, 1994.

Meola T, Soter NA, Ostreicher R, et al: The safety of UVB phototherapy in patients with HIV infection. *J Am Acad Dermatol* 29:216, 1993.

Odom RB, Berger TG: The cutaneous manifestation of AIDS. *Curr Concepts* 1:32, 1990.

Pardo RJ, Bogaert MA, Penneys NS, et al: UVB phototherapy of the pruritic papular eruption of the acquired immunodeficiency syndrome. *J Am Acad Dermatol* 26:423, 1992.

Penneys NS: *Skin Manifestations of AIDS*. London, Dunitz, 1990.

Schlesinger I, Oelrich DM, Tyring SK: Crusted (Norwegian) scabies in patients with AIDS: The range of clinical presentations. *South Med J* 87:352, 1994.

Impetigo

Background   **Evaluation**
Etiology   **Treatment**
Clinical Presentation

Background

Impetigo is a common cutaneous bacterial infection that primarily affects children. This superficial infection usually is caused by *Streptococcus pyogenes* (group A β-hemolytic streptococci) or *Staphylococcus aureus*. It may occur as a primary condition or secondarily complicate preexisting dermatoses such as atopic dermatitis, varicella, and scabies. Impetigo classically is divided into bullous and nonbullous forms. The bullous form is almost exclusively caused by *S. aureus*.

Etiology

There are two necessary conditions for the appearance of impetigo in a patient. First, the patient must be colonized by the pathogenic organism. Neither *S. aureus* nor *S. pyogenes* is part of the normal skin flora. Acquisition of the pathogenic organism may be from affected family members or close personal contacts. Crowding and poor personal hygiene are known risk factors for the development of impetigo. For *S. pyogenes,* spread to a previously unaffected individual occurs in the skin first, with subsequent spread to the respiratory tract. In contrast, *S. aureus* initially colonizes the nasal mucosa and may be isolated from the skin approximately 11 days later.

The second condition necessary for the development of impetigo is a break in the skin. As a rule, intact skin is resistant to impetiginization. The disruption of the normal skin may be due to minor trauma such as abrasions and insect bites. Alternatively, preexisting dermatoses such as atopic dermatitis, varicella, and scabies may disrupt the normal cutaneous barrier. Once infection occurs, the resultant inflammation is superficial, with vesicopustules located between the stratum corneum and the stratum granulosum.

Escherichia coli, Peptostreptococcus, Prevotella, Fusobacterium, Bacteroides fragilis, and other bacteria may occasionally be responsible. Most organisms that cause impetigo produce the enzyme ß-lactamase.

Bullous impetigo virtually always is due to *S. aureus.* The bullae result from an exotoxin produced by *S. aureus,* most commonly group II phage type 71, which results in subcorneal epidermal cleavage.

Clinical Presentation

Impetigo is more common in hot humid climates, with a peak incidence in late summer and early fall. Although it is seen in all age groups, children 2 to 5 years of age are the most commonly affected. The lesions often appear rapidly, and a history of previous minor trauma to the affected area often can be elicited. Pain generally is not noted although pruritus is an occasional complaint. Fever and systemic symptoms are rare. If it is untreated, new lesions may continue to appear, but the disease is generally self-limited with resolution over 2 to 3 weeks.

Nonbullous impetigo initially presents as a thin-walled vesicle on an erythematous base that quickly progresses to a pustule. These vesicles and pustules rupture easily, leaving the characteristic "honey-colored" or yellow-brown crust over the superficial erosion (Figs. 10-1 through 10-4). Occurrences are most common on the extremities and face, particularly in periorificial locations. The initial lesions are usually not larger than 1 or 2 cm, but larger areas may become involved through coalescence of lesions. Regional lymphadenopathy is present in most of these patients. With time, the lesions may heal centrally, giving the clinical appearance of a dermatophyte infection. Healing occurs without scarring.

Bullous impetigo initially demonstrates large flaccid bullae on an erythematous base. However, because these lesions are so fragile, a superficial erosion with a thin crust and collarette of scale is often all that is seen on initial presentation. Regional lymphadenopathy is less common than it is in nonbullous impetigo. As with nonbullous impetigo, over time the lesions may heal centrally, giving the clinical appearance of a dermatophyte infection. Healing occurs without scarring.

Figure 10-1

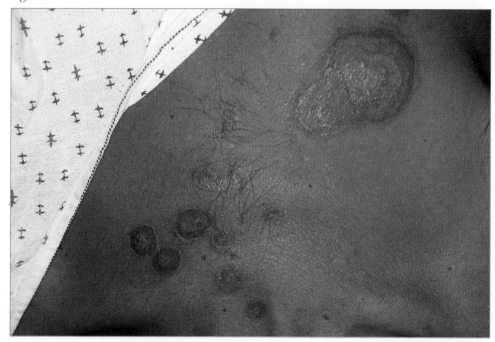

Crusting and erythema associated with acute impetigo.

Complications of impetigo are uncommon but may include progression to deeper infections such as ecthyma and cellulitis. Impetigo caused by streptococcal species may rarely be followed by scarlet fever or, more significantly, acute poststreptococcal glomerulonephritis. After the impetigo, a latent period of 18 to 21 days precedes the onset of the glomerulonephritis. Unfortunately, antibiotic treatment of streptococcal impetigo does not prevent the development of glomerulonephritis. Similarly, rheumatic fever also can rarely occur as a result of streptococcal skin infections. Clinicians should be aware of these potential complications.

Evaluation

Generally, the diagnosis is evident from the typical appearance of the lesions. Bacterial culture with antibiotic sensitivities may be performed as antibacterial therapy is empirically initiated. These results may be used to guide changes in therapy if

Figure 10-2

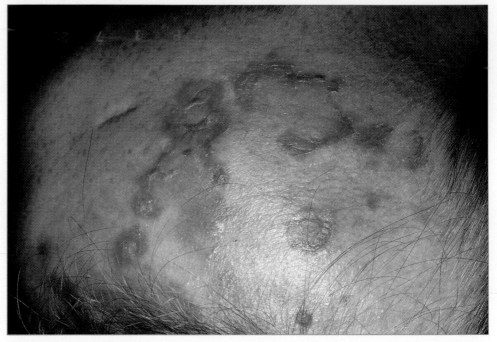

Large patches of impetigo.

the empirical treatment is not effective. Biopsy is rarely indicated but may be useful in atypical cases.

Treatment

Although impetigo, if left untreated, generally resolves on its own within 2 to 3 weeks, treatment will prevent the lesions from becoming more numerous and hasten recovery. For patients with uncomplicated localized disease, the use of topical mupirocin (Bactroban) three times a day for 7 to 10 days has been found to be as effective as oral erythromycin. It is effective against the most frequent skin pathogens, including those resistant to other antibiotics, and topical administration allows the delivery of high drug concentrations to the site of infection. Topical treatment does not prevent rheumatic fever, though skin infection with streptococci almost never causes rheumatic fever.

For more extensive involvement in which the clinician feels that topical therapy is likely to miss some lesions, the use of systemic antibiotics is recommended. Since

S. aureus is often present with or without coinfection with *S. pyogenes,* ß-lactamase-resistant antibiotics should be used for 7 to 10 days. These oral agents include dicloxacillin, cephalexin, amoxicillin with clavulanic acid (Augmentin), erythromycin, and azithromycin. Factors affecting antibiotic choice include cost and patterns of antibiotic resistance in the clinician's area.

Patients with multiple recurrent cases are likely to be chronic nasal carriers of *S. aureus.* Eradication of this carrier state may be accomplished through the application of mupirocin to the nares twice daily for 1 week each month. Alternatively, treatment with a systemic antistaphylococcal antibiotic combined with rifampin 300 mg twice per day in an adult is generally effective. Rifampin may also be added to any antibiotic regimen when the patient does not respond to therapy.

In areas of high prevalence, application of topical antibiotics prophylactically to children in sites of minor trauma may reduce the frequency of impetigo. While good hygiene may help prevent spread, treatment with antibiotics is the main means by which the potential for contagion is reduced. When treatment appears ineffective, culture for sensitivity of the organism may be helpful. Often, culture will show that the offending organism is sensitive to the antibiotic that has been prescribed, indicating the possibility of treatment failure caused by poor adherence to the treatment regimen.

Figure 10-3

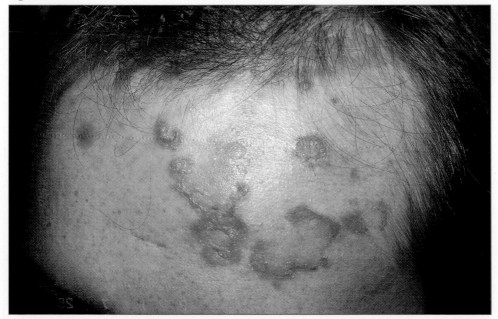

The face is a common impetigo location.

Figure 10-4

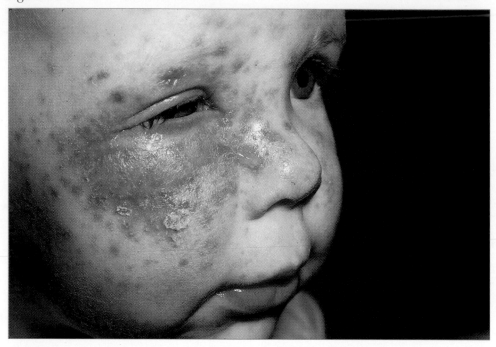

Children with crusting and exudate may be highly contagious.

Bibliography

Barnett BO, Frieden IJ: Streptococcal skin diseases in children. *Semin Dermatol* 11:3, 1992.

Brook I, Frazier EH, Yeager JK: Microbiology of nonbullous impetigo. *Pediatr Dermatol* 14:192, 1997.

Dagan R: Impetigo in childhood: Changing epidemiology and new treatments. *Pediatr Ann* 22:235, 1993.

Darmstadt GL, Lane AT: Impetigo: An overview. *Pediatr Dermatol* 11:293, 1994.

Feder HM Jr, Pond KE: Addition of rifampin to cephalexin therapy for recalcitrant staphylococcal skin infections—an observation. *Clin Pediatr* 35:205, 1996.

Feingold DS: Staphylococcal and streptococcal pyodermas. *Semin Dermatol* 12:331, 1993.

Hogan P: Paediatric dermatology: Impetigo. *Aust Fam Phys* 27:735, 1998.

Kahn RM, Goldstein EJ: Common bacterial skin infections: Diagnostic clues and therapeutic options. *Postgrad Med* 93:175, 1993.

Kobayashi S, Ikeda T, Okada H, et al: Endemic occurrence of glomerulonephritis associated with streptococcal impetigo. *Am J Nephrol* 15:356, 1995.

Leyden JJ: Review of mupirocin ointment in the treatment of impetigo. *Clin Pediatr* 31:549, 1992.

Sadick NS: Current aspects of bacterial infections of the skin. *Dermatol Clin* 15:341, 1997.

Scales JW, Fleischer AB Jr, Krowchuk DP: Bullous impetigo. *Arch Pediatr Adolesc Med* 151:1168, 1997.

Shriner DL, Schwartz RA, Junniger CK: Impetigo. *Cutis* 56:30, 1995.

Chapter 11

Tinea and Superficial Fungal Infections

Background

More than 100,000 species of fungi have been identified worldwide, but 5 or 6 of those species account for most dermatophytoses globally. Since tinea infections with these organisms are a universal human experience, familiarity with the latest concepts in diagnosis and treatment can help clinicians care for patients with these infections.

Epidemiology

Tinea infection is one of the most common dermatologic reasons for patients to see a primary care provider. The incidence of tinea capitis is declining in many nations, while tinea pedis and onychomycosis are becoming more common. Tineas affect both men and women, but in adulthood they are more common in men. Tinea capitis is more common in the black population. The reason for this is unknown, although both social and genetic factors have been suggested.

Dermatophytes are contagious. Dissemination of dermatophytes depends on direct or indirect contact between infected and uninfected hosts. In this process, colonization of the epidermal stratum corneum is the first step. The infectious component of the dermatophyte is most likely to be the arthrospore or a hyphal fragment adhering to or contained in a corneocyte. The increased use of athletic shoes by both men and women and communal bathing could be contributing factors to the increase in tinea pedis. Fomites such as combs and hats may play a role in the spread of tinea capitis.

Pathophysiology

On the basis of their primary habitats, dermatophytic organisms may be grouped as geophilic (soil-associated), zoophilic (animal-associated), and anthropophilic (human-associated). Although infections with any organism itch, zoophilic and geophilic species are more likely to be inflammatory and itchy. Most of the infectious agents of the dermatophytoses are classified in three genera: *Epidermophyton, Microsporum,* and *Trichophyton. Trichophyton rubrum* is the most common cause worldwide of tinea pedis, nail infection, tinea cruris, and tinea corporis. Pityriasis, or tinea versicolor, is not a tinea but is caused by an overgrowth of the normal skin inhabitant *Malassezia furfur (Pityrosporum orbiculare).*

Dermatophytes grow in the nonliving cornified layer of keratinized tissue (skin, hair, and nails); they do not penetrate viable tissue of an immunocompetent host. The presence of dermatophytes elicits a host response that ranges from mild to severe. Acid proteinases, elastase, keratinases, and other proteinases reportedly act as virulence factors.

The development of cell-mediated immunity correlated with delayed hypersensitivity and an inflammatory response is associated with clinical cure, whereas the lack of or defective cell-mediated immunity predisposes the host to chronic or recurrent dermatophyte infection. Even if immunity develops, certain dermatophytes, such as *T. rubrum,* produce substances that diminish the immune response.

The immune response probably helps control clinical infections. Some individuals may be relatively more susceptible to infection than are others; thus, the infection is more likely to gain a "toehold." The factors that underlie this susceptibility are poorly understood. In regard to this issue, the use of potent topical or systemic corticosteroid agents may inhibit the immune response, encouraging the growth of dermatophytes.

Clinical Features

Tinea infections are named according to the body location affected: feet, tinea pedis; groin, tinea cruris; hand, tinea manuum; face, tinea faciei; body, tinea corporis; scalp, tinea capitis; and nails, tinea unguium. Within each location, tinea infections vary widely in appearance. Clinically, the typical appearance of most dermatophyte infections is a scaling ring on any part of the body (Fig. 11-1), but a wide variety of other morphologies exist, including scaling patches, plaques, hyperpigmented patches and plaques, and bullous lesions.

Figure 11-1

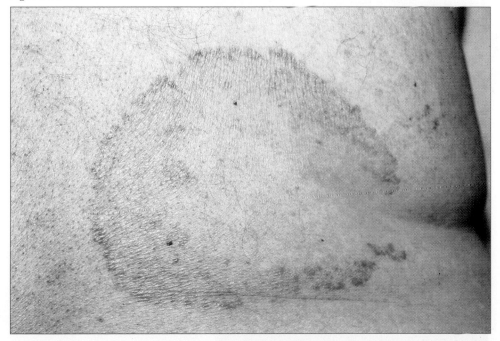

While both tinea and dermatitis are red and scaly, tinea infections tend to have an outer scaly ring with central clearing.

The symptoms of tineas are also variable. Inflammatory tineas and other superficial fungi may be strikingly itchy, but many tineas are not itchy because the organisms cause little host response. Patients may question the diagnosis of tinea because they are not experiencing any symptoms from the eruption.

At times, the inflammatory response to tinea infections may be extensive, including boggy, inflamed, draining kerion reactions in the scalp. Autoeczematization and generalized itchy "dermatophytid" reactions may occur; these terms refer to itchy dermatitic involvement of uninfected skin. The most common of these "id" reactions is an itchy dermatitic eruption of the hands in patients with severely inflamed tinea pedis.

Tinea Pedis (Athlete's Foot)

Tinea pedis is a foot dermatophyte infection that is most commonly caused by *T. rubrum* and less commonly caused by *T. interdigitalis* and *E. floccosum*. Interdigital infections of dermatophytes may result in maceration and leukokeratosis of the interdigital space (Figs. 11-2 and 11-3), with overgrowth of various bacteria, including *Micrococcus sedantarius, Brevibacterium epidermidis, Corynebacterium*

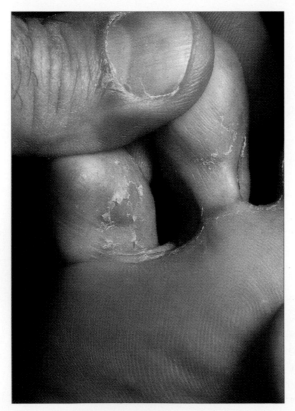

Figure 11-2

Interdigital tinea pedis. The scaling without maceration seen here represents the early stage of interdigital tinea infection. The fourth web space is the most common area of involvement. Involvment of this area is helpful in distinguishing fungal infection from a contact dermatitis (e.g., contact dermatitis to leather or rubber in shoes tends to spare the web space).

Figure 11-3

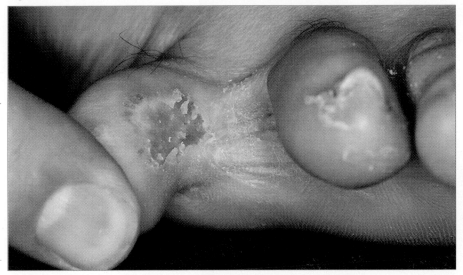

Interdigital tinea pedis. The maceration in this well-developed lesion is a common component of interdigital tinea infection. (From Fitzpatrick TB et al: *Color Atlas and Synopsis of Clinical Dermatology, 3/e.* New York, McGraw-Hill, 1995, p. 693.)

minutissimum, and gram-negative organisms. A moccasin type of hyperkeratosis in which the entire sole is covered by diffuse scaling is usually due to *T. rubrum* (Fig. 11-4). Vesiculobullous infections in the arch and the side of the foot result from an immune response to *T. mentagrophytes.* Erythema and scaling only of the weight-bearing surfaces, sparing the webs, are more suggestive of an eczematous process than of tinea.

Tinea Cruris (Jock Itch)

Tinea cruris is most commonly caused by *T. rubrum* or *E. floccosum* (Fig. 11-5). The groin is a moist place that serves as a veritable culture plate for fungal growth. A well-demarcated erythematous brown to brown patch or plaque with a superficial scale is typical. The edge may or may not be more inflamed than is the center.

Tinea Corporis (Ringworm)

Tinea corporis is a dermatophyte infection of the major skin surfaces. In hot and humid areas, tinea corporis is more common and usually is caused by *T. rubrum.* The appearance usually includes pink to red patches and plaques with central clearing and scale (Fig. 11-6), and the sharp margin helps differentiate the eruption from atopic or xerotic dermatitis. Zoophilic dermatophytes such as *M. canis,*

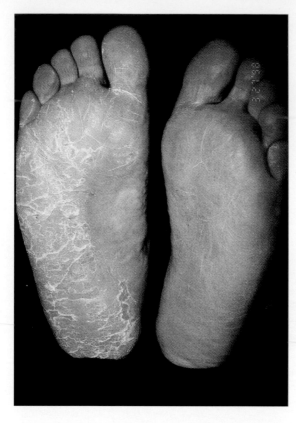

Figure 11-4

Moccasin-type involvement of the entire foot with tinea. The sharp cutoff at the borders of the plaque favors tinea over dermatitis, though a KOH examination is needed to differentiate these conditions.

Figure 11-5

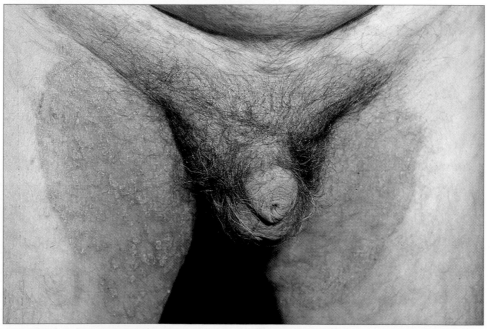

Tinea cruris must be differentiated from intertrigo (intertriginous dermatitis). The sharp margins indicate tinea cruris. A KOH examination is confirmatory of tinea infection. (From Fitzpatrick TB et al: *Color Atlas and Synopsis of Clinical Dermatology, 3/e.* New York, McGraw-Hill, 1995, p. 699.)

Figure 11-6

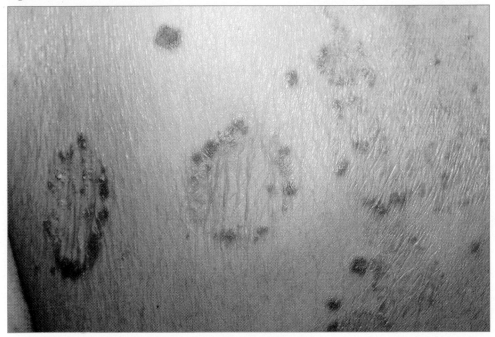

Annular rings with central clearing are typical of tinea corporis.

and *T. verrucosum* may occur after the appropriate animal exposure and are likely to be highly inflammatory. A common scenario in children is occurrence in siblings after exposure to a new kitten or puppy obtained from an animal shelter. In adults with extensive tinea corporis, diabetes may be a predisposing factor.

Tinea Capitis

Tinea capitis is a fungal infection of the scalp with invasion of the hair shafts by a dermatophyte. Dermatophytes that typically cause tinea capitis include *M. canis, M. audouinti,* and *T. tonsurans.* Clinically, one sees a patch of alopecia with the black dots of hairs that are broken (Figs. 11-7 and 11-8). Follicular pustules also are evident. When there is extreme inflammation, a nodular lesion called a kerion may be seen.

Tinea Faciei and Tinea Barbae

Tinea of the face may exhibit three distinct patterns. There may be red, scaly lesions similar to those seen in tinea corporis (Fig. 11-9); we refer to this as tinea faciei. Tinea faciei often is confused with lupus erythematosus and other inflammatory facial eruptions. Often, these eruptions are not recognized as tinea and are

Figure 11-7

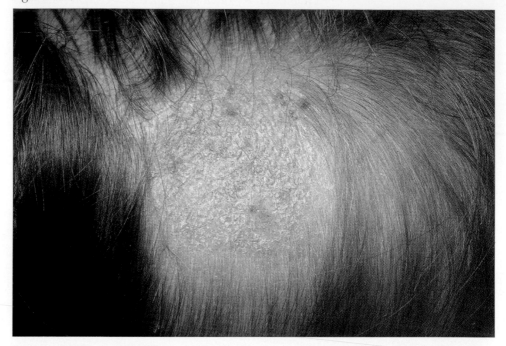

Hair loss in a well-delineated patch with scaling or small "black dots" is indicative of tinea capitis.

Figure 11-8

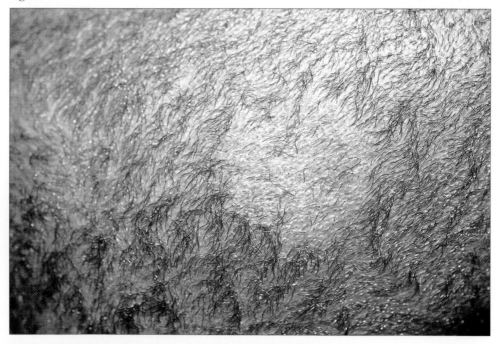

Tinea capitis is most common in blacks and in the pediatric age group.

Figure 11-9

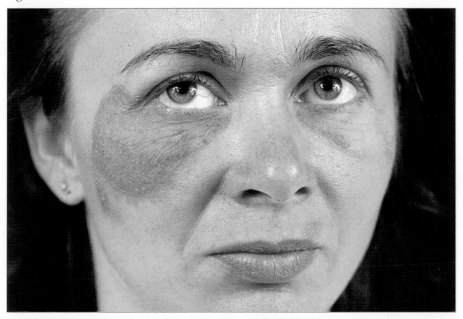

Tinea faciei. Tineas of the face often are mistaken for other inflammatory diseases and are treated with topical corticosteroids. This can result in an atypical presentation (less scaling and central clearing). Identification of a sharp margin and performance of a KOH examination make the diagnosis. (From Fitzpatrick TB et al: *Color Atlas and Synopsis of Clinical Dermatology, 3/e.* New York, McGraw-Hill, 1995, p. 703.)

Figure 11-10

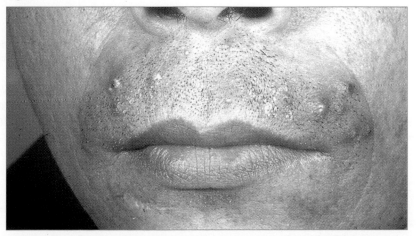

Tinea barbae, folliculitis type. (From Fitzpatrick TB et al: *Color Atlas and Synopsis of Clinical Dermatology, 3/e.* New York, McGraw-Hill, 1995, p. 710.)

Figure 11-11

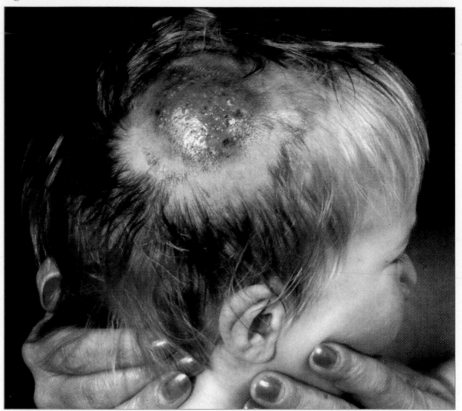

Tinea barbae, kerion type. Kerion infections are large boggy masses studded with pustules. (From Fitzpatrick TB et al: *Color Atlas and Synopsis of Clinical Dermatology, 3/e*. New York, McGraw-Hill, 1995, p. 707.)

treated with topical corticosteroids, with subsequent spread. Recognition of the sharp borders and confirmatory potassium hydroxide (KOH) examination make the diagnosis.

The two other forms occur in the beard area, are similar to the forms of tinea capitis, and are refered to as tinea barbae. In tinea barbae, lesions range from multiple pustules resembling bacterial folliculitis (Fig. 11-10) to a markedly inflammatory type resembling a kerion (Fig. 11-11).

Tinea Manuum

Tinea manuum is a dermatophyte infection of the palms that most commonly is due to *T. rubrum*. Typically, there is a diffuse chronic scaling of the palms. Often it is diagnosed as eczema or psoriasis; this is unfortunate, as tinea manuum flourishes in the presence of topical corticosteroids. Vesicles occasionally are seen. A common presentation is "one-hand, two-foot tinea" in which bilateral tinea pedis accompanies unilateral tinea manuum.

The incidence of tinea manuum should not be exaggerated. Compared to hand dermatitis, tinea manuum is quite rare. Unless there is marked involvement of the feet, dermatitic-appearing eruptions of the hands are almost universally hand dermatitis, not a tinea infection.

Tinea Unguium (Onychomycosis)

Tinea unguium is a fungal infection of the nails that is most commonly caused by *T. rubrum*. Chronically moist toenails make an excellent fungal culture medium. Fungi most commonly invade from the distal end (distal subungual onychomycosis). Tinea infections of the nails are uncommon in younger people, who have a fairly rapid growth rate of the nails, but become more common after the fifth decade. The nail appears to be thickened and crumbling and to have subungual debris (Fig. 11-12). Nail fungal infections are caused not only by dermatophytes but also by yeasts such as *Candida* and saprophytes such as *Hendersonula* and *Scopulariopsis*.

Figure 11-12

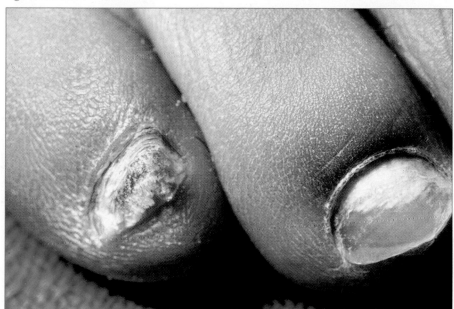

The most common form of onychomycosis is distal subungual onychomycosis, as seen on the left. A less common form is superficial white onychomycosis, as seen on the right. Treatment of onychomycosis is effective only if oral antifungal therapy is used. Onychomycosis must be differentiated from psoriatic nail dystrophy. A positive KOH examination can demonstrate the presence of onychomycosis; the presence of psoriatic lesions elsewhere generally is indicative of psoriatic nail dystrophy.

Figure 11-13

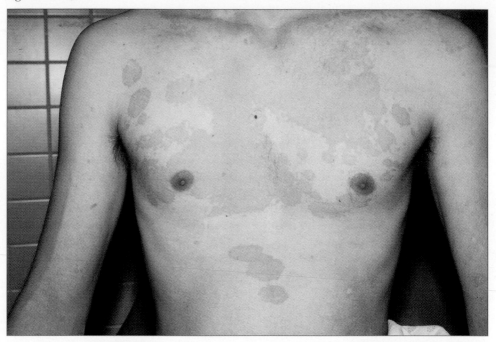

Tinea versicolor generally exhibits diffuse involvement of the trunk, although it may be localized and present in other areas.

Tinea Versicolor (Pityriasis Versicolor)

Tinea versicolor is caused by *Pityrosporum orbiculare*. *Pityrosporum* is a normal skin organism. When it grows exuberantly, there are well-demarcated hypo- or hyperpigmented scaling patches typical of tinea versicolor (Figs. 11-13 through 11-15). These lesions are typically on the anterior and posterior chest but can occur over much of the body surface. Although they are hyperpigmented on pale skin, when the surrounding skin suntans, the areas of tinea versicolor are usually paler than the surrounding skin.

Laboratory Confirmation

While tinea infections can be strongly suspected on the basis of characteristic clinical findings, laboratory tests are helpful in confirming the diagnosis. The primary test is the KOH preparation. Although there are no definite guidelines on when to perform a KOH test, the old adage "If it scales, scrape it" is a fairly good guide.

Samples of skin lesions are obtained by using a number 15 blade or glass slide to scrape scale from the advancing edge of a lesion. The sample is placed on a microscope slide, and KOH 10 to 20% is added under a coverslip. Branching hyphae (Fig. 11-16) can be visualized with light microscopy, using a stopped-down condenser to obtain contrast. Nail specimens are collected in the same manner.

Culture of scrapings is helpful if the KOH smear is negative and a tinea is strongly suspected. Culture is a more sensitive technique, especially in the setting of onychomycosis, since much more material can be examined. Mycosel or Sabouraud agar is used occasionally and allows for identification of fungal species. Dermatophyte test medium (DTM) also may be used but does not allow speciation. Speciation is generally not neccesary for guiding treatment; similarly, antifungal sensitivity testing generally is used for research and not clinical purposes. The samples for fungal culture are obtained in the same fashion as in the KOH preparation.

If a KOH preparation and fungal culture are not positive and a fungal etiology is still suspected, a skin biopsy can be done. A periodic acid-Schiff (PAS) stain helps visualize hyphae in the stratum corneum. Biopsy is generally not a first-line diagnostic technique because of the added cost, pain, and scarring.

When lesions involve the scalp, a Wood's lamp can be used to detect fluorescence found with species of *Microsporum*. This technique is not as valuable as it

Figure 11-14

Scattered scaly hypopigmented lesions of the trunk are strongly suggestive of tinea (pityriasis) versicolor.

Figure 11-15

Slight redness and scaling are common in the lesions of tinea versicolor.

once was, as most tinea capitis now is caused by *T. tonsurans,* an organism that does not fluoresce.

Treatment

General Measures

Treatment is directed at changing the environment that encourages the growth of dermatophytes. Suggestions to patients may include completely drying the skin after bathing, allowing a full day for shoes to dry between uses, changing socks during the day, intermittent prophylactic use of over-the-counter topical antifungals, and the use of appropriate drying powders (cornstarch should be avoided, as it may encourage fungal growth; a powder containing miconazole may be the most helpful).

Figure 11-16

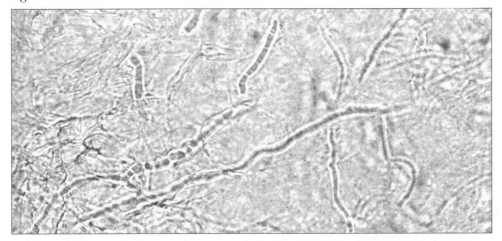

A positive KOH examination. Branching septate hyphae are shown here. Often, far fewer organisms are seen in the specimen. (From Fitzpatrick TB et al: *Color Atlas and Synopsis of Clinical Dermatology, 3/e.* New York, McGraw-Hill, 1995, p. 691.)

Topical Agents

Topical treatment with topical antifungal agents is indicated for limited body surface areas and incidents when the infection does not involve the nails or hair (that is, in limited forms of tinea corporis, tinea pedis, tinea cruris, and tinea faciei). Systemic treatment, as described below, is needed for extensive infection and when the hair or nails are involved. A summary of the most commonly used types of medications and their use in different conditions is presented in Tables 11-1 and 11-2. As a general rule, the cream should be applied to the symptomatic area as well as 1 or 2 cm beyond the visible eruption. Treatment should continue for a week after resolution of the visible rash. There are advantages to using broad-spectrum agents such as the azoles for superficial fungal infections. Clinicians should remember that nystatin has robust activity against yeasts such as *Candida* but has no activity against dermatophytes.

For skin involved with tinea versicolor, topical therapy is appropriate for both large and small areas of infection. Selenium sulfide 2.5% lotion may be applied to large areas, avoiding the nipples and genitalia, and washed off in the morning. Selenium sulfide may be irritating to sensitive skin. A recently introduced alternative for large-area topical treatment is terbinafine spray. Oral ketoconazole also has been used. Although ketoconazole rarely causes hepatotoxicity, this approach may be prefered by some patients because of its convenience. In cases where tinea versicolor presents with a limited focal eruption, topical use of an azole cream product is effective and appropriate.

Table 11-1

Topical and Systemic Antifungal Agents

TYPE OF AGENT	EXAMPLES	ADVANTAGES	DISADVANTAGES
		TOPICAL AGENTS	
Azoles	Miconazole, clotrimazole (in many OTC products), sulconazole (Exelderm), oxiconazole (Oxistat), econazole (Spectazole)	Broad spectrum of activity against dermatophytes and yeasts	Few
Allylamines	Naftifine (Naftin), terbinafine (Lamisil)	Highly effective against dermatophytes	Less effective against yeasts
		SYSTEMIC AGENTS	
Azoles	Itraconazole (Sporanox), fluconazole (Diflucan), ketoconazole (Nizoral)*	Broad spectrum of activity against dermatophytes and yeasts	Many drug interactions; potential for hepatoxicity
Allylamines	Terbinafine (Lamisil)	Generally most effective agent against dermatophytes	Less effective against yeasts; rare cause of systemic side effects
Griseofulvin	Griseofulvin (Grifulvin)	Generally safe; may be treatment of choice for pediatric tinea capitis	Many drug interactions, though rarely a problem in the pediatric (tinea capitis or corporis) population; minor side effects (headache and gastrointestinal upset common); marginal efficacy for onychomycosis

* Ketoconazole is less effective that the other oral azoles and no longer is recommended as an oral therapy for true tinea infections.

Systemic Treatments

Systemic treatments are used for hair infection (tinea capitis and barbae), nail infection (onychomycosis), and extensive tinea infections (e.g., extensive tinea corporis or moccasin-type tinea pedis). Details of the systemic treatments are described below; general guidelines are presented in Table 11-2. Tinea capitis in children may be treated with griseofulvin. Terbinafine is the treatment of choice for onychomycosis. Either agent may be used for extensive tinea corporis or moccasin-type tinea pedis.

Table 11-2

Treatment Options for Different Forms of Tinea Infection

INFECTION	FIRST-LINE TREATMENT	SECOND-LINE TREATMENT
Localized tinea of glabrous skin (pedis, cruris)	Topical azole cream (bid for 2 weeks generally adequate)	Oral griseofulvin or terbinafine for refractory disease
Extensive tinea corporis or moccasin-type tinea pedis	Oral terbinafine (500 mg/d for 2 to 4 weeks)	Oral terbinafine (250 mg/d for 1 to 2 weeks)
Tinea capitis	Oral griseofulvin (20 mg/kg per day of microsized for 6 weeks)	Oral terbinafine (125 mg/d for 4 weeks)
Onychomycosis	Terbinafine (250 mg/d for 3 months)	Itraconazole (200 mg bid for 1 week a month for 3 months)
Tinea versicolor	Selsun 2.5% lotion weekly for 3 weeks, then at 3- to 6-month intervals to prevent recurrence	Ketoconazole 400 mg orally daily for 3 months; repetition at intervals is necessary to treat recurrences

GRISEOFULVIN

Tinea capitis requires treatment with a systemic antifungal such as griseofulvin. Griseofulvin microsized is available in suspension and should be given to children at 15 to 20 mg/kg per day for 4 to 6 weeks. Tablet or capsule forms of griseofulvin microsized (15 to 20 mg/kg per day) or ultramicrosized (6 mg/kg per day) are also available. The side effects of griseofulvin include gastrointestinal upset, headaches, and numerous drug interactions, including with warfarin, barbiturates, and cyclosporine. Laboratory monitoring usually is not necessary. Because of its safety profile and high efficacy, griseofulvin remains the treatment of choice for children with tinea capitis. Griseofulvin also can be used for extensive or treatment-resistant tinea corporis (10 mg/kg per day for 4 weeks), but other agents in adults, such as terbinafine, are superior.

Griseofulvin is no longer a drug of choice for onychomycosis. Because it has poor affinity for keratin, griseofulvin must be used until the infection clears. In the scalp, this may take 1 to 5 months.

TERBINAFINE

Terbinafine is an allylamine that has been found to be effective and safe in therapy for dermatophyte infections. It is not as effective as azole antifungal agents in treating candidiasis but is the most effective agent in treating dermatophytes.

Terbinafine usually is given to adults in doses of 250 mg orally a day for 5 days (tinea versicolor), 6 weeks (onychomycosis of the fingernails), or 12 weeks (onychomycosis of the toenails). In adults, a 2-week course of terbinafine 250 mg/d is generally sufficient to clear tinea pedis, cruris, and corporis. There is not a specified dose for the treatment of tinea capitis in children who are resistant to griseofulvin, but terbinafine may prove to be the agent of choice for this indication. This agent generally has fewer side effects and fewer drug interactions than do other systemic antifungal medications. Rare side effects include hepatotoxicity and pancytopenia. If therapy continues with terbinafine for more than 6 weeks, liver transaminases should be monitored.

ITRACONAZOLE

Itraconazole is a broad-spectrum triazole that has been found to be effective and safe in brief therapy for dermatophyte infections. This medication is used for the treatment of a variety of fungal infections. Often, two 400-mg doses are sufficient to cure the yeast infection pityriasis (tinea) versicolor. For tinea unguium in adults, a regimen of 200 mg bid given in a pulse fashion 1 week of each month for 3 months versus a daily dose of 200 mg/d is used. This approach is not as effective against dermatophytosis of the nails but may be more effective in treating saprophytes and *Candida*.

Ongoing studies with tinea capitis may help determine the role of this agent in treating griseofulvin-resistant disease. Itraconazole is significantly less effective than terbinafine in treating dermatophyte nail infections. Side effects include possible hepatotoxicity and multiple, potentially serious drug interactions with agents such as astemizole, cisapride, cyclosporine, digoxin, and warfarin. Liver transaminases should be monitored before therapy and periodically throughout the therapy if the therapy lasts for more than 1 month.

FLUCONAZOLE

Fluconazole also belongs to the class of triazoles and has been studied primarily in candidiasis. In candidiasis, it appears to be an excellent and well-tolerated agent. Very little information has been published on its efficacy in dermatophyte infections, and so it may not be a treatment of choice. Studies of efficacy in nail infections suggest that fluconazole is approximately as effective as itraconazole and markedly less effective than terbinafine. Until further information is available, the other agents listed above may be better choices in treating dermatophyte infections.

Bibliography

Aly R: Ecology and epidemiology of dermatophyte infections. *J Am Acad Dermatol* 31:S21, 1994.

Bergus GR, Johnson JS: Superficial tinea infections. *Am Fam Phys* 48:259, 1993.

Brodell RT, Elewski B: Superficial fungal infections: Errors to avoid in diagnosis and treatment. *Postgrad Med* 101:279, 1997.

Brooks KE, Bender JF: Tinea pedis: Diagnosis and treatment. *Clin Podiatr Med Surg* 13:31, 1996.

Dahl MV: Suppression of immunity and inflammation by products produced by dermatophytes. *J Am Acad Dermatol* 28:S19, 1993.

Degreef HJ, DeDoncker PR: Current therapy of dermatophytosis. *J Am Acad Dermatol* 31:S25, 1994.

Elewski BE, Hazen PG: The superficial mycoses and the dermatophytes. *J Am Acad Dermatol* 21:655, 1989.

Fleischer AB Jr: *The Clinical Management of Itching.* New York, Parthenon, 1988.

Leyden JJ, Aly R: Tinea pedis. *Semin Dermatol* 12:280, 1993.

McClean DL, Sober SJ: *Illustrated Dermatology.* Advanstar Communications, Inc., and Lasion Europe NV, 1994.

Rezabek GH, Friedman AD: Superficial fungal infections of the skin: Diagnosis and current treatment recommendations. *Drugs* 43:674, 1992.

Richardson MD: Diagnosis and pathogenesis of dermatophyte infections. *Br J Clin Pract* 71:98, 1990.

Roberts DT: Oral terbinafine (Lamisil) in the treatment of fungal infections of the skin and nails. *Dermatology* 194 (Suppl 1):37, 1997.

Silva-Lizama E: Tinea versicolor. *Int J Dermatol* 34:611, 1995.

Weitzman I, Summerbell RC: The dermatophytes. *Clin Microbiol Rev* 8:240, 1995.

Chapter

12

Varicella Zoster Virus Infections

Background

Varicella zoster virus (VZV) is a double-stranded DNA virus of the human herpes virus family. Primary infection with VZV leads to a generalized exanthem known as varicella (chickenpox) and accounts for 3.5 million cases annually in the United States. Exposure to VZV is nearly universal in the United States, with more than 90 percent of adults having serologic evidence of prior infection. With the recent advent of the varicella vaccine, the proportion of the population with serologic evidence of antibodies probably will be even higher. The virus subsequently sets up a latent infection in the sensory nerve ganglia and may reactivate later in life as herpes zoster (shingles). Herpes zoster accounts for another 300,000 cases of VZV per year and affects over 10 percent of the total population over their lifetimes.

Etiology

For primary VZV infection (i.e., clinical or subclinical varicella), no gender or racial differences are known. Children are primarily affected, with over 90 percent of cases occurring by age 14. In the United States, varicella epidemics tend to occur in the winter and spring.

Transmission of VZV is accomplished mainly via airborne droplets, with the initial infection probably occurring in the upper respiratory tract. It also may be possible to aquire varicella through direct physical contact with an infectious host. Varicella is highly contagious, with the attack rate in susceptible persons after exposure being about 87 percent. Herpes zoster also produces airborne viral particles, and the viral infection may be transmitted without physical contact.

Several types of exposure can place susceptible persons at risk for varicella. Direct contact exposure is defined as more than 1 h of direct contact with an infectious person while indoors. Brief contacts with an infectious person are less likely to result in VZV transmission than are more prolonged contacts. Persons with continuous exposure to household members who have varicella are at the greatest risk for infection. Varicella develops in approximately 90 percent of susceptible household contacts.

After initial viral replication at the initial site of infection, viremia occurs. At some time during the primary infection, the virus invades sensory nerve fibers and travels to sensory nerve ganglia, where it establishes latent infection, usually in a dermatome innervated by the sensory nerve. Subsequent alterations in host factors may allow for virus reactivation in which the virus multiplies and spreads down the affected nerve, leading to clinical lesions in a dermatomal pattern.

Clinical Presentation

Varicella

Varicella has an incubation period of about 2 weeks between exposure to an infectious individual and the onset of symptoms. Cutaneous lesions may be preceded by a 2- to 3-day prodrome of low-grade fever, chills, malaise, arthralgias, myalgias, and anorexia. Initially, erythematous maculopapules are seen, which subsequently progress to small vesicles on an erythematous base, to pustules, and then to crusted lesions (Figs. 12-1 and 12-2). The lesions are often extremely pruritic. The cutaneous eruption tends to begin on the head or trunk, with subsequent centripetal spread. New lesions tend to occur in crops and may be noted for the first 4 days,

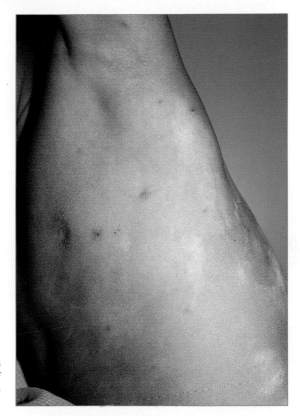

Figure 12-1

A widespread eruption of erythematous macules and vesicles in different stages of evolution. This boy presented after the application of calamine lotion.

with subsequent crusting and healing of lesions over 2 weeks. Classically, lesions at all stages of progression may be seen simultaneously on the same patient. Patients should be evaluated for evidence of secondary infection of the lesions. Patients should be considered contagious from 2 days before the rash appears until all the lesions have crusted.

Any person who has not been vaccinated or had an active infection is susceptible. In one study, a history of previous varicella infection in adults with varicella was found not to be reliable. True second episodes of varicella probably are rare in immunocompetent adults.

The most commonly seen complication of varicella is secondary infection of the cutaneous lesions with subsequent scarring. More serious complications include Reye's syndrome in children and varicella pneumonitis in adults. Reye's syndrome (fatty liver with encephalopathy) has been linked to aspirin use in patients with varicella. Varicella pneumonitis develops in about 1 percent of adults with primary varicella, with an increased risk in pregnant women and the immunocompromised.

Neonatal varicella is seen when maternal varicella occurs from 5 days before to 2 days after delivery. It frequently is associated with visceral complications and significant mortality. Fetal varicella syndrome may rarely occur, with maternal

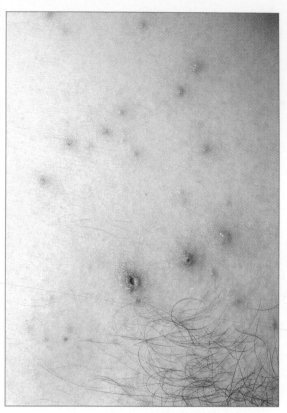

Figure 12-2

Close-up view of umbilicated vesicles typical of varicella virus infection.

varicella occurring at 8 to 20 weeks of gestation. The syndrome is characterized by limb hypoplasia, cortical atrophy, cutaneous scars, and other anomalies.

Herpes Zoster

The incidence of herpes zoster increases with advancing age and immunocompromise of various etiologies [human immunodeficiency virus (HIV) infection, immunosuppressive medications, and malignancy]. The initial symptoms of herpes zoster are often pain and paresthesia in the affected dermatome. The pain usually precedes the cutaneous eruption by 2 to 3 days. Thoracic dermatomes are the most commonly affected, followed by lumbar and trigeminal dermatomes. Constitutional symptoms, including malaise and lethargy, are not common.

The cutaneous eruption most frequently consists of closely grouped vesicles on an erythematous base and goes through the same stages of evolution that were noted above for varicella. The lesions are unilateral, do not cross the midline, and generally are limited to one or two continuous dermatomes (Figs. 12-3 through 12-6). A significant number of patients may have several vesicles outside the affected dermatome, presumably as a result of hematogenous dissemination. Lymphadeno-

Figures 12-3

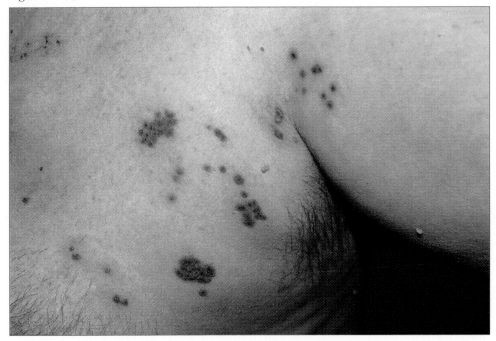

Dermatomal zoster in adults with typical vesicles.

pathy, is noted frequently. Complete resolution of the lesions usually occurs in 2 to 3 weeks.

When zoster involves the face, careful examination for lesions on the tip of the nose is important, as these lesions indicate involvement of the nasociliary branch of the ophthalmic division of the trigeminal nerve, which also innervates the eye. Thus, zoster on the nose tip indicates a risk for ocular involvement.

It is recognized that zoster may manifest as dermatomal paresthesias or dysesthesias without a cutaneous eruption. Similarly, a motor nerve may be involved, with resultant temporary or permanent paralysis. This motor nerve involvement is particularly problematic when it involves extraocular muscles, leading to diploplia, or facial muscles, leading to facial droop.

The most common complications of herpes zoster are secondary infection of the cutaneous lesions with subsequent scarring and postherpetic neuralgia.

Postherpetic neuralgia (PHN) is defined as pain that persists after complete healing of the cutaneous eruption. Risk factors for PHN include increasing age, severe pain, and trigeminal distribution. More than 50 percent of zoster patients over 60 years old develop PHN, which may persist for months, years, or decades. PHN accounts for about 15 percent of all referrals to pain clinics. Clinicians can make a difference, as antiviral treatment may have some effect in reducing the incidence of PHN.

Figure 12-4

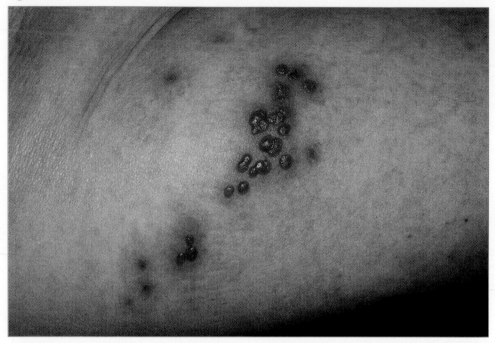

Dermatomal zoster in adults with typical vesicles.

Figure 12-5

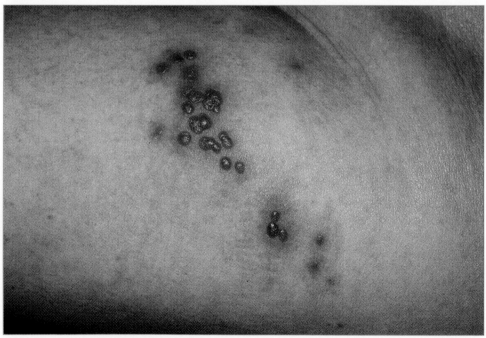

Dermatomal zoster in adults with typical vesicles.

Figure 12-6

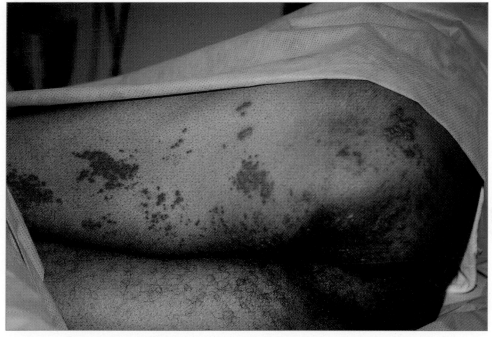

Dermatomal zoster in adults with typical vesicles.

Other, less common complications include corneal scarring and visual loss caused by involvement of the ophthalmic division of the trigeminal nerve (herpes zoster ophthalmicus) and unilateral facial nerve palsy (Ramsay Hunt syndrome).

Evaluation

The diagnosis of varicella or herpes zoster usually is made on the basis of a typical history and physical examination. To confirm the suspected diagnosis and in cases with atypical presentations, the following additional tests may be helpful.

A Tzanck smear of a vesicular lesion may be performed rapidly in the office and should demonstrate multinucleate giant cells (Fig. 12-7). This technique requires a great deal of training, and methods of performing Tzanck smears are beyond the scope of this book. A Tzanck smear will not differentiate herpes simplex virus (HSV) from herpes zoster.

Viral culture may be performed and is capable of differentiating HSV-1, HSV-2, and VZV. The best results are obtained when the test is performed on vesicular lesions. However, VZV is notoriously difficult to grow in culture.

Direct fluorescent antibody (DFA) stain of infected cells scraped from ulcerated lesions may be performed. Biopsy may be suggestive of VZV infection and is

Figure 12-7

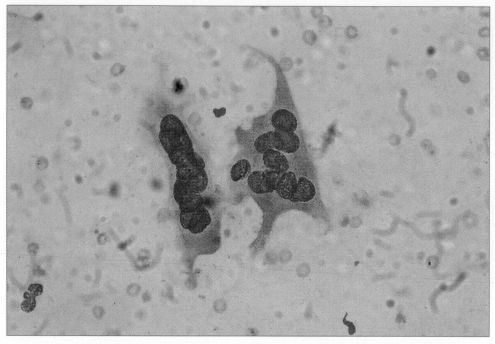

Examination of vesicle fluid reveals characteristic multinucleated giant cells.

useful to rule out other conditions. Biopsy interpretation cannot distinguish HSV from VZV unless immunoperoxidase staining for VZV is performed. The polymerase chain reaction test, where clinically available, is the most sensitive technique for identifying VZV DNA.

Treatment

Prevention of VZV Infection

LIVE ATTENUATED VARICELLA VACCINE

In 1995, a live attenuated varicella vaccine was approved by the U.S. Food and Drug Administration. The recommended age for vaccination of children is 12 to 18 months. The vaccine is administered as a 0.5-mL subcutaneous dose to children age 1 to 12 years who have not had chickenpox. Those over age 12 should receive two 0.5-mL subcutaneous doses 1 to 2 months apart.

Table 12-1

Contraindications to VZV Vaccination

History of anaphylactoid reaction to neomycin
Immunocompromised patients
High-dose immunosuppressive therapy
Moderate or severe illness
Pregnancy and breast-feeding
Having received immune globulin or varicella zoster immune globulin within the preceding 5 months
Blood transfusion within the preceding 5 months

These regimens provide 70 to 90 percent protection against infection and 95 percent protection against severe disease. When breakthrough cases occur, they are generally milder, with fewer than 50 lesions. Because the vaccine is a live attenuated virus, vaccine recipients still are at risk for developing herpes zoster infections later in life from the vaccine strain. Contraindications to vaccination are listed in Table 12-1.

It has been hypothesized that the varicella vaccine also may be useful in preventing zoster in older adults with waning cellular immunity. Although the vaccine may play a major role in this regard in the future, there have been no controlled trials. Immunocompromised children and adults also may benefit from the vaccine in preventing the potentially serious complications that arise as a result of infection or reactivation. However, because this is a live virus vaccine, profoundly immunocompromised hosts, such as patients with advanced HIV disease, may be at risk of serious vaccine-related disease.

VARICELLA-ZOSTER IMMUNE GLOBULIN

Varicella-zoster immune globulin (VZIG) is a parenteral, intramuscularly administered globulin fraction of human plasma, primarily immunoglobulin G. It is used for passive immunization of immunocompromised patients after exposure to chickenpox or herpes zoster. The recommended regimen has been shown to modify the severity of chickenpox and reduce the frequency of death, pneumonia, and encephalitis compared with no therapy.

According to the Centers for Disease Control and Prevention (CDC), the decision to administer VZIG to a person exposed to varicella should be based on (1) whether the patient is susceptible either by having a negative history of varicella or by lacking documentation of vaccination, (2) whether the exposure is likely to result in infection, and (3) whether the patient is at greater risk for complications than is the general population. The use of the VZIG generally should decline as the varicella vaccine gains wider acceptance and use. An example of a situation in which use of this agent may be appropriate is a profoundly immunosuppressed acquired immunodeficiency syndrome (AIDS) patient with no history of chickenpox or shingles who has close personal contact with someone who has an acute

VZV infection. Contraindications include an allergic response to gamma globulin, anti-immunoglobulin A antibodies, and thimerosal.

The dosage in adults is to administer within 96 h after exposure 125 units/10 kg injected deep intramuscularly (IM). Doses should be given in multiples of 125 units (2.5 mL), with no more than 250 units at a single site. The maximum dose is 625 units. For primary prophylaxis in HIV-infected patients with no history of chickenpox or shingles, the CDC recommends a dose of 5 vials (12.5 mL) injected deep IM, administered ±96 h after exposure but ideally within 48 h. In immuno-compromised children or infants, the CDC recommends 1 vial (1.25 mL)/10 kg (maximum of 5 vials) IM within 96 h after exposure, ideally within 48 h. Pregnant women should be evaluated in the same manner as other adults; however, because such women are at higher risk for severe varicella and complications, VZIG should be strongly considered for susceptible pregnant women who have been exposed. The use of VZIG in other patients should be judged on a case-by-case basis and should take into account a patient's susceptibility, the extent of exposure, and the likelihood of complications.

Varicella Treatment

SYMPTOMATIC THERAPY

Although only a small percentage of patients with primary varicella infection develop severe complications from the disease, the vast majority of patients are quite miserable with this disease. Symptomatic therapy with or without specific antiviral therapy is therefore important in all patients.

The fever most patients develop usually responds well to antipyretics such as ibuprofen and acetaminophen. Salicylates should be avoided because of potential risk of Reye's syndrome. For most patients, the most bothersome symptom is the intense pruritus of the lesions. Systemic sedating antihistamines such as diphenhydramine and hydroxyzine are often helpful. Additionally, tepid baths with or without colloidal oatmeal (Aveeno) may temporarily ameliorate the pruritus. As a result of the intense pruritus, patients often cause deep excoriations, leading to secondary bacterial infection and scarring. If there is any sign of secondary infection, the use of topical antibiotic preparations such as mupirocin (Bactroban) may be helpful.

ANTIVIRAL THERAPY

The use of acyclovir (Zovirax) in healthy children and adults has been shown to modestly reduce the total number of lesions, the duration of fever, and the duration of illness compared with placebo. Systemic acyclovir clearly decreases disease duration and may allow parents to return to work sooner. Given the proven safety of acyclovir, the use of this agent can be strongly recommended. Some experts suggest that the routine use of acyclovir in children remains somewhat controversial and advocate only symptomatic therapy for otherwise healthy children. These experts maintain, without convincing evidence, that natural immunity acquired without treatment may be more robust. Furthermore, they state that the cost

Table 12-2

Varicella Zoster Therapy for Patients

PATIENT GROUP	DRUG	DOSE AND DURATION
Healthy adults	Acyclovir	800 mg orally 5 times a day for 7 days
	Famciclovir	500 mg orally 3 times a day for 7 days
	Valacyclovir	1000 mg orally 3 times a day for 7 days
Healthy children	Acyclovir	20 mg/kg orally 4 times a day for 7 days
Immunocompromised adults	Acyclovir	10 mg/kg intravenously every 8 h for 7–10 days
Immunocompromised children	Acyclovir	500 mg/m^2 intravenously every 8 h for 7–10 days

of the agent is unjustified. There is little debate, however, regarding the use of acyclovir in immunocompromised patients with varicella, in whom it is clearly indicated. The best responses are achieved when therapy is initiated within 24 h of the onset of the rash. The dosing schedules for acyclovir are shown in Table 12-2.

Famciclovir (Famvir) and valacyclovir (Valtrex) are useful alternatives to acyclovir. Neither agent is available in a suspension form, and so their use in young children is difficult. Famciclovir and valacyclovir have distinct advantages over acyclovir. Both are more readily absorbed when administered orally and may be used less often to achieve the same effect. Until proven efficacious and safe, neither agent should be used in immunocompromised patients.

Herpes Zoster Treatment (Fig. 12-8)

SYMPTOMATIC THERAPY

As with patients with primary varicella infection, patients with herpes zoster are frequently miserable. However, for these patients, pain, not pruritis, is the major symptom. Although nonsteroidal anti-inflammatory drugs and acetaminophen may be tried, frequently these patients may require other analgesics, including narcotics, to control the pain. The use of narcotic analgesic agents for limited periods often is greatly appreciated by patients in pain.

Cool compresses may be helpful in ameliorating the pain. In patients for whom pruritus is a major symptom, treatment such as that for varicella may be used. These treatments include systemic sedating antihistamines and topical antibiotics to prevent or treat secondary bacterial infection.

ANTIVIRAL THERAPY

Several studies have shown that immunocompetent patients with herpes zoster benefit from antiviral therapy. Patients receiving antiviral therapy have a shorter duration of acute illness as well as decreased severity and duration of pain. Some studies also suggest a benefit for the prevention of PHN. Other studies have shown an unclear benefit for antiviral therapy. Given the severity of PHN and the limited toxicity of the antiviral agents, antiviral therapy generally is advocated. For all treatment regimens, benefits are most likely to be noted if therapy is started within 2

Figure 12-8

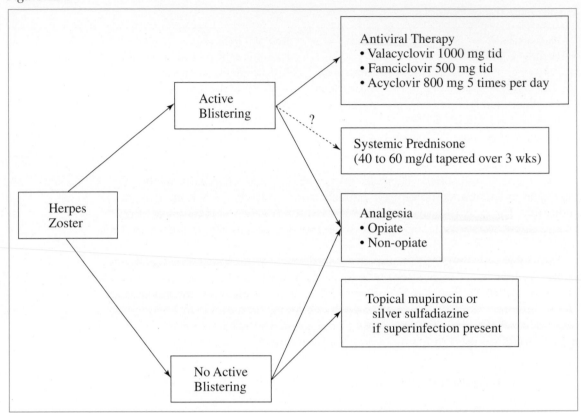

Algorithm for the treatment of herpes zoster.

days of the onset of the rash. The treatment regimens for the various antiviral medications in adults are listed in Table 12-2. Famciclovir and valacyclovir are preferable to acyclovir because these agents require fewer daily doses and are often less expensive than acyclovir.

Immunocompromised patients with herpes zoster also benefit from antiviral therapy. Treatment with acyclovir has been shown to prevent cutaneous dissemination and limit visceral involvement. Treatment with valacyclovir should be avoided in immunocompromised patients because of the occurrence of thrombotic thrombocytopenic purpura and the hemolytic-uremic syndrome in these patients during clinical trials. Until more information is available, famciclovir should be avoided in this special population. The dosing of acyclovir for immunocompromised patients is described in Table 12-2.

CORTICOSTEROID THERAPY

The use of systemic corticosteroid therapy is controversial in herpes zoster patients. Before effective antiviral therapy became available, they were widely used to decrease acute pain and reduce the severity of PHN. In the present era of effective antiviral therapy, there is no convincing evidence that they can play a special role in treating herpes zoster. Corticosteroids plus acyclovir did not provide an added benefit over acyclovir alone in one study, but this combination did appear to improve the quality of life of older patients in another investigation. Similar studies have not been performed with the more effective agents valacyclovir and famciclovir. Accordingly, clinicians should decide whether they will add corticosteroids to an antiviral regimen.

Studied regimens included prednisone (60 mg/d for the first 7 days, 30 mg/d for days 8 to 14, and 15 mg/d for days 15 to 21) and prednisolone (initiated at 40 mg/d and tapered over a 3-week period). Systemic corticosteroid agents produce acute side effects, particularly in the elderly population treated for this indication. Some clinicians routinely prescribe systemic corticosteroid agents in combination with antiviral therapy, whereas others do not. The data remain unclear about the best course of action regarding steroid administration.

AMITRIPTYLINE

Amitriptyline (25 mg/d) was studied in a randomized, double-blind, placebo-controlled trial for 90 days after the initial diagnosis of zoster. The results showed that early treatment with amitriptyline reduced acute and chronic pain prevalence by more than one-half. This suggests that there may be a role for the preemptive administration of amitriptyline in combination with an antiviral drug to elderly patients with acute herpes zoster.

Amitriptyline has numerous side effects, ranging from postural hypotension and urinary retention to xerostomia. Accordingly, its benefits in the elderly population need to be weighed against its side effects. It is unclear whether other antidepressant medications are as efficacious as amitriptyline.

POSTHERPETIC NEURALGIA

Patients over age 50 are particularly at risk for the development of PHN, which can be excruciatingly painful and notoriously difficult to treat. This may present as burning, itching, or pain in the original distribution of the vesicles and seems to be due to nerve damage from the virus and the inflammatory response to the virus. In the vast majority of patients, the symptoms are gone within 2 months. Some patients may retain pain, however, for months to years.

The systemic tricyclic antidepressant medication amitriptyline (Elavil), initially at a dose of 25 mg hourly and slowly increasing to 100 mg hourly, may be the most effective known medication for this condition. It has been shown repeatedly in controlled trials to be efficacious, whereas other therapies have not withstood this scrutiny. Treatment with amitriptyline may take several weeks until a significant reduction in pain is noted.

Preemptive treatment with low-dose tricyclic antidepressant agents at the time of onset of zoster (amitriptyline or nortriptyline 10 to 25 mg hourly) reduces the incidence of PHN by about half. Established PHN should be treated with tricyclic agents over 2 or 3 weeks in doses up to 100 mg/d.

Topical capsaicin (Zostrix) applied three to five times daily may play an adjunctive role. This agent theoretically depletes substance P and other neuromodulators from sensory nerves, leading to decreased pain sensations. This medication may induce severe burning sensations on the skin, and so patients should begin using the medication cautiously and wash the hands thoroughly after application. Treatment with capsaicin may take several weeks until a significant reduction in pain is noted.

Other pharmacologic agents have been tried and have advocates in the treatment of PHN, ranging from carbamazepam to gabapentin. Unfortunately, there are very few trials suggesting efficacy for many agents. If these approaches do not prove effective, the clinician should consider referral to a specialized clinic for pain management. A multidisciplinary approach ranging from counseling to nerve blocks can help patients with intractable pain.

Bibliography

AMA Council on Scientific Affairs: Immunization of health care workers with varicella vaccine. *J Okla State Med Assoc* 90:376, 1997.

Arvin AM: Varicella-zoster virus: Overview and clinical manifestations. *Semin Dermatol* 15:4, 1996.

Bowsher D: The effects of pre-emptive treatment of postherpetic neuralgia with amitriptyline: A randomized, double-blind, placebo-controlled trial. *J Pain Sympt Manag* 13:327, 1997.

Bowsher D: The management of postherpetic neuralgia. *Postgrad Med J* 73:623, 1997.

Brody MB, Moyer D: Varicella-zoster virus infection: The complex prevention-treatment picture. *Postgrad Med* 102:187, 1997.

Choo PW, Galil K, Donahue JG, et al: Risk factors for postherpetic neuralgia. *Arch Intern Med* 157:1217, 1997.

Erlich KS: Management of herpes simplex and varicella-zoster virus infections. *West J Med* 166:211, 1997.

Gershon AA: Epidemiology and management of postherpetic neuralgia. *Semin Dermatol* 15 (Suppl 1):8, 1996.

Haanpaa M, Hakkinen V, Nurmikko T: Motor involvement in acute herpes zoster. *Muscle Nerve* 20:1433, 1997.

Herne K, Cirelli R, Lee P, Tyring SK: Antiviral therapy of acute herpes zoster in older patients. *Drugs Aging* 8:97, 1996.

Jackson JL, Gibbons R, Meyer G, Inouye L: The effect of treating herpes zoster with oral acyclovir in preventing postherpetic neuralgia: A meta-analysis. *Arch Intern Med* 157:909, 1997.

Johnson CE, Stancin T, Fattlar D, et al: A long-term prospective study of varicella vaccine in healthy children. *Pediatrics* 100:761, 1997.

Johnson RW: Herpes zoster and postherpetic neuralgia: Optimal treatment. *Drugs Aging* 10:80, 1997.

MacFarlane LL, Sanders ML, Carek PJ: Concerns regarding universal varicella immunization: Time will tell. *Arch Fam Med* 6:537, 1997.

Prevention of varicella: Recommendations of the Advisory Committee on Immunization Practices (ACIP): Centers for Disease Control and Prevention. *MMWR* 45:1, 1996.

Sawyer MH, Chamberlin CJ, Wu YN, et al: Detection of varicella-zoster virus DNA in air samples from hospital rooms. *J Infect Dis* 169:91, 1994.

Tyring SK: Efficacy of famciclovir in the treatment of herpes zoster. *Semin Dermatol* 15:27, 1996.

Varicella-related deaths among adults—United States, 1997. *MMWR* 46:409, 1997.

Ventura A. Varicella vaccination guidelines for adolescents and adults. *Am Fam Phys* 55:1220, 1997.

Volmink J, Lancaster T, Gray S, Silagy C: Treatments for postherpetic neuralgia—A systematic review of randomized controlled trials. *Fam Pract* 13:84, 1996.

Wallace MR, Chamberlin CJ, Zerboni L, et al: Reliability of a history of previous varicella infection in adults. *JAMA* 278:1520, 1997.

Whitley RJ, Kimberlin DW: Treatment of viral infections during pregnancy and the neonatal period. *Clin Perinatol* 24:267, 1997.

Whitley RJ, Weiss H, Gnann JW Jr, et al: Acyclovir with and without prednisone for the treatment of herpes zoster: A randomized, placebo-controlled trial. *Ann Intern Med* 125:376, 1996.

Wood MJ, Johnson RW, McKendrick MW, et al: A randomized trial of acyclovir for 7 days or 21 days with and without prednisolone for treatment of acute herpes zoster. *New Engl J Med* 330:896, 1994.

Warts

Background

Warts are benign epithelial proliferations of the skin and mucous membranes caused by infection with one of many varieties of the human papillomavirus (HPV). These lesions also are known as verrucae, papillomas, and condylomata. This chapter focuses on warts as a dermatologic problem, including common, flat, and plantar warts. Treatment options for external genital warts also are covered. Cervical and anal HPV infection is beyond the scope of this chapter.

Epidemiology

Warts in any location may be found in persons of all ages, from neonates to the elderly. Nongenital warts are found more commonly in children and young adults, with the peak incidence in the teenage years. Anogenital warts usually are found in sexually active patients. Warts in anogenital areas may be spread by both sexual and nonsexual means. Individuals with impaired cell-mediated immunity, such as patients taking cyclosporine and those infected with the human immunodeficiency virus, are much more susceptible to warts and are usually more resistant to treatment. The rare hereditary immunodefieciency epidermodysplasia verruciformis also causes massive wart proliferation.

As many as half of all sexually active adults have been infected with HPV, but only a small minority display visible warts. The infectivity of subclinically infected patients is unknown.

Pathophysiology

The human papillomaviruses are a family of double-stranded DNA viruses that are host-specific (human HPV does not infect other animals, and HPV of other animals does not infect humans). There are several hundred types of HPV, and certain types have an affinity for a specific body location, such as the foot or the mucous membranes. A subclass of HPV has a malignant potential and may be found in certain cervical carcinomas. Transmission of HPV depends on many factors, including host susceptibility, the quantity of infectious virus present, and the location of lesions. The virus is inoculated into the epithelium through defects in the epidermis. The viral genome resides in epithelial cells, and a clinically detectable wart develops 2 to 9 months later. Autoinoculation to other sites is common.

Clinical Features

Warts are usually chronic and slow-growing. Most patients are distressed more by the appearance of warts than by the associated symptoms. However, secondary irritation in pressure-bearing locations such as the feet may produce significant pain or tenderness. Warts may bleed easily if traumatized. Genital warts may itch.

Common Warts (Verruca Vulgaris)

Common warts are hyperkeratotic papules or plaques that appear steep-shouldered. Often thrombosed vessels appear as tiny black dots within the wart. They can occur on any skin surface, especially the hands, fingers, knees, and other points of trauma, and may be grouped (Figs. 13-1 through 13-3). Some lesions have a filiform appearance.

Flat Warts (Verruca Plana)

Flat warts are more flat-topped and less hyperkeratotic than common warts. They may appear flesh-colored or have brown tones (Figs. 13-4 and 13-5). They usually are found as grouped lesions on the face, or on the legs of women who shave.

Plantar Warts

Plantar warts, which are found on the bottom of the feet, may appear similar to a callus or corn, but the "black dots" (which represent thrombosed capillaries) within a wart can enhance this differentiation (Fig. 13-6). Mosaic warts are large hyperkeratotic plaques, usually found on the plantar surface of the feet, that result from

Figure 13-1

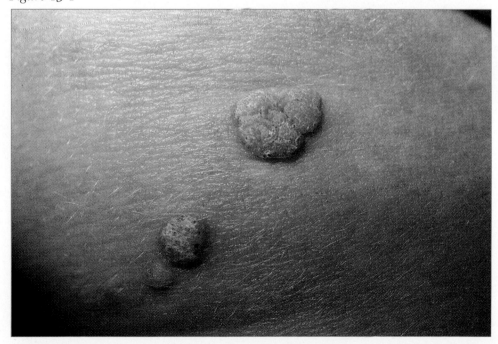

Grouped common warts.

Figure 13-2

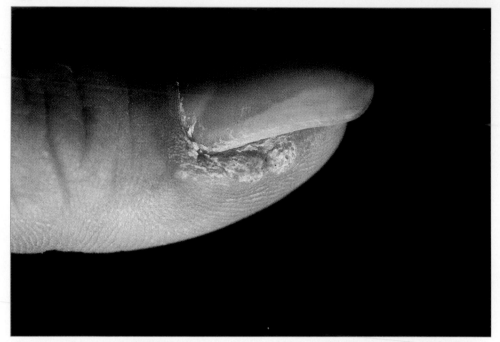

Periungual warts are a challenge to remove.

Figure 13-3

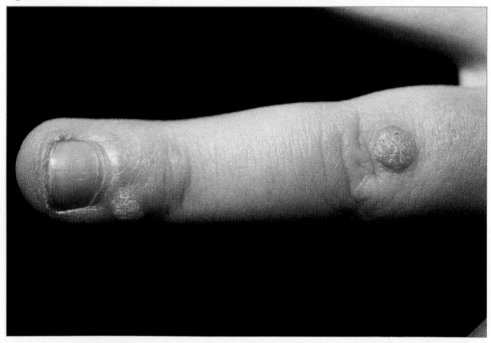

Common warts occur frequently in children and teenagers. The finger is a commonly affected area.

Figure 13-4

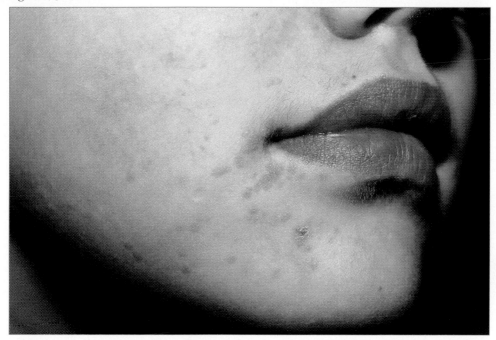

Flat warts occur most commonly on the face and legs. Shaving may contribute to the spread of the lesions.

Figure 13-5

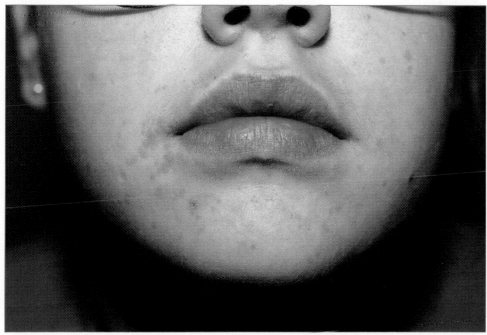

Flat warts.

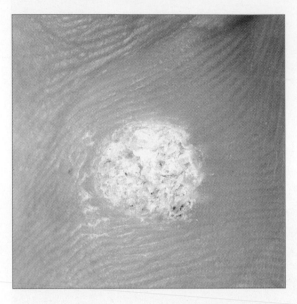

Figure 13-6

Plantar wart. The thromboses capillaries (black dots) in the wart help differentiate this lesion from a callus (clavus). (From Fitzpatrick TB et al: *Color Atlas and Synopsis of Clinical Dermatology, 3/e.* New York, McGraw-Hill, 1995, p. 769.)

the coalescence of multiple smaller warts. Unlike common warts that grow "out," plantar warts appear to grow "in" because of the pressure of walking on them. The wart becomes like a foreign object the patient is standing on and can be quite painful.

Anogenital Warts (Condyloma Acuminata)

Anogenital warts appear as hyperkeratotic or dermal flesh-colored papules in the genital or perianal mucosa. These lesions vary in size from 1-mm papules to large (10 by 10 cm), exophytic cauliflower-like masses (Fig. 13-7, *A* through *C*). Bowenoid papulosis consists of erythematous to hyperpigmented warty papules on the external genitalia. Although they have the clinical appearance of warts, these papules exhibit histologic features of squamous cell carcinoma in situ. These lesions usually result from infection with HPV-16 and other oncogenic viruses and may be a precursor to penile or vulvar carcinoma.

Evaluation

Warts generally are diagnosed by clinical appearance, but the diagnosis also can be made by histopathologic examination of skin biopsy specimens. This may be necessary in sun-exposed areas of older patients to distinguish the lesion (e.g., a cutaneous horn) from a keratoacanthoma, actinic keratosis, or squamous cell

Figure 13-7

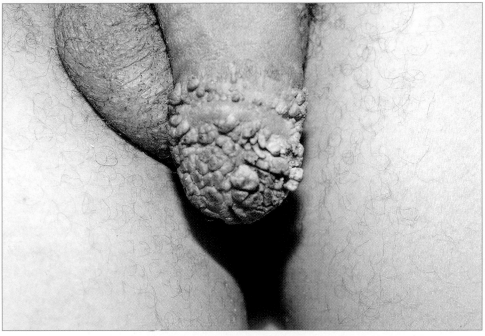

a

Genital warts may be flat, papular, or cauliflower-like, with the latter termed condyloma accuminata.

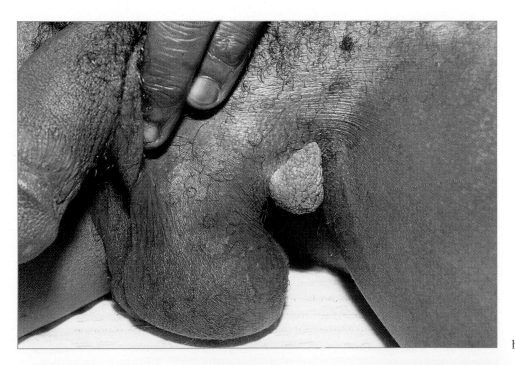

b

Figure 13-7 (Continued)

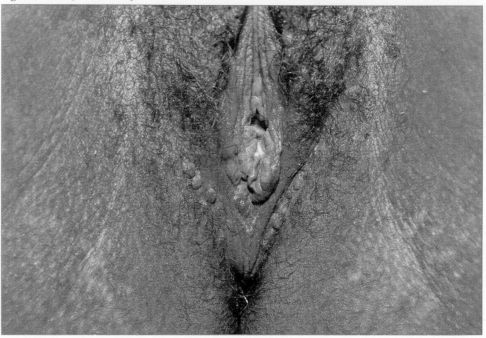

c

The moist texture of the skin in this area allows the penetration of topical agents, making podophylin and imiquimod more effective than they are in other areas.

carcinoma. Immunohistochemical or DNA hybridization techniques can be performed to identify the type of HPV that is present. This is rarely, if ever, necessary for diagnosis or treatment.

In the male genitalia, accentuating the difference between normal and diseased skin with acetic acid has proponents. Acetowhite lesions are identified by means of the topical application of 5% aqueous acetic acid. Unfortunately, this technique has high false-positive rates, and there has never been a study demonstrating enhanced remission periods in patients who employ this technique. Accordingly, the value of acetowhite application is unproven.

Complications

Rarely, preexisting warts may develop into low-grade squamous cell carcinomas. This occurs in the oral cavity (florid oral papillomatosis), anogenital area (giant condyloma of Buschke-Lowenstein), and plantar surface of the foot (epithelioma cuniculatum). Women and sexual contacts of male patients being treated for condyloma acuminata should consider a thorough gynecologic examination to rule out cervical involvement. Some authors recommend that men and women with extensive perianal lesions undergo proctoscopic examination.

With the exception of the few problems cited above, most of the complications from wart disease stem from the complications of treating warts, including infection and scarring. For instance, urethral stricture may result from chemical or mechanical destruction in the urethral area. Accordingly, the side effects of treatment should always be considered before treatment initiation.

Treatment

The approach to the management of warts takes many factors into consideration, including the patient's desire for treatment, the age and immune status of the patient, and the size and location of the lesion or lesions. We teach patients that "treatment of warts is a process, not an event." Patients and/or their parents often request laser therapy or other intensive measures for treating warts. Because some interventions are painful and costly and may induce scarring, it is prudent to make sure the merits of a treatment modality outweigh the side effects.

Patients present with folk beliefs regarding treatments and amusing anecdotes. The clinician should bear in mind that all warts in patients with normal immune systems will resolve spontaneously if given enough time. Harmless and ineffective treatments such as homeopathic remedies appeal to a subpopulation of patients.

Most medical treatments involve the destruction of infected epithelial cells. Topical agents, which may be used in combination with liquid nitrogen cryotherapy, are usually the first-line therapy. Resistant lesions may respond to procedures such as electrodesiccation and laser therapy. The commonly used treatments for warts are discussed below. There are no definite guidelines, but a general approach for different lesions is described in Tables 13-1 and 13-2. None of the treatments is universally effective, and the cure rates for the different treatments are not well characterized, and so the treatment approach has great latitude. Wart treatment can be frustrating at times; perseverance usually results in good outcomes, but therapy should not be so intense as to be worse than the disease.

Topical Therapy

ACIDS

SALICYLIC OR LACTIC ACID   Initial topical therapy for common warts may consist of salicylic or lactic acid solutions or plasters, which usually can be obtained over the counter. These acids act as "keratolytics" to break up the thick scale on the surface of the wart; this therapy is most useful for warts that have thick scale on their surface, as is commonly seen in plantar warts. Treatment of plantar warts with these preparations can be considered successful if the wart resolves or if a painful wart is converted to an asymptomatic wart.

Table 13-1

Treatment Options for Warts in Children

Common warts: single or few lesions	1. Cryotherapy, if child tolerates pain
	2. If not tolerated, topical cantharidin to the lesion(s) may be effective
	3. Surgery [electrodessication and/or curettage (ED&C), excision, or laser] only if highly symptomatic
Common warts: numerous lesions	1. Watchful waiting for 3 months
	2. Cryotherapy to most bothersome lesions if tolerated; topical cantharidin to lesions if cryotherapy is not tolerated
	3. Topical imiquimod daily under occlusion
	4. Surgery (ED&C, excision, or laser) only if highly symptomatic
Flat warts	1. Cryotherapy, if tolerated for limited number of lesions
	2. Topical tretinoin (0.025% gel) 1 to 2 times a day for 3 months
Plantar warts	1. Daily use of topical salicylic acid preparation and home debridement (may be continued indefinitely as long as patient remains asymptomatic)
	2. Gentle debridement to remove thick scale, followed by cryotherapy if tolerated
	3. Surgical removal (ED&C, excision, or laser) only if highly symptomatic and refractory to other treatments
Genital warts	1. Evaluation for possible sexual abuse (genital warts in children do not necessarily imply sexual abuse)
	2. Topical imiquimod 3 times a week for up to 16 weeks
	3. Cryotherapy, if tolerated for a few lesions

The keratolytic preparations are applied daily after soaking the wart to increase penetration. The choice of solution or plaster generally is based on patient preference. The wart can be debrided at home in the mornings with either a blade or an emery board after overnight application of the keratolytic. If this treatment is not successful after 6 to 8 weeks, an additional treatment modality may be required. Some clinicians prefer to apply this agent themselves.

TRICHLOROACETIC ACID   Trichloroacetic acid (TCA) is a destructive therapy. It can be used for any wart type, but some feel that it is more useful for the treatment of anogenital warts. It is applied in the office carefully by the clinician, using a cotton applicator.

PODOPHYLLIN

Podophyllin is a topical solution that is more effective for the treatment of anogenital warts. The 20 to 50% solution usually is applied in the clinician's office

Table 13-2

Treatment Options for Warts in Adults

Common warts: single or few lesions	1. Cryotherapy 2. Surgery [electrodessication and/or curettage (ED&C), excision, or laser] only if highly symptomatic
Common warts: numerous lesions	1. Cryotherapy 2. Immunotherapy 3. Interferon therapy only if highly symptomatic 4. Surgery (ED&C, excision, or laser) only if highly symptomatic
Flat warts	1. Avoidance of spreading by shaving 2. Cryotherapy to worst lesions plus topical retinoic acid (0.025% gel) 1 to 2 times a day for 3 months
Plantar warts	1. Daily use of topical salicylic acid preparation and home debridement (may be continued indefinitely as long as patient remains asymptomatic) 2. Gentle debridement to remove thick scale, followed by cryotherapy 3. Surgical removal (ED&C, excision, or laser) only if highly symptomatic and refractory to other treatments
Genital warts	1. Evaluation for other sexually transmitted diseases 2. Cryotherapy or trichloroacetic acid destruction for few lesions 3. Podophyllotoxin (Condylox) bid to lesions 3 days a week for 4–8 weeks or office application of 20% podophyllin for 1–6 weeks (women respond better) 4. Topical imiquimod (Aldara) 3 times a week for up to 16 weeks (women respond better)

and is washed off by the patient with soap and water after 4 to 6 h. Care is taken to allow the solution to dry so that the podophyllin does not spread to an unaffected area. Up to six consecutive treatments may be required for complete resolution of the warts. The use of podophyllin is contraindicated during pregnancy.

PODOPHYLLOTOXIN (CONDYLOX)

Podophyllotoxin 0.5% is a purified derivative of podophyllin. It is available in solution and gel vehicles and may be applied twice daily for 3 consecutive days per week to genital warts for 1 to 3 months. The advantage of this approach is that fewer office visits are required to bring the warts to resolution, and many patients prefer this approach over office podophyllin or cryotherapy. The disadvantage is that only about two-thirds of women and only one-third of men respond completely. Accordingly, it should be considered one of many options in dealing with genital warts. When side effects occur, patients experience burning, stinging, and pain.

TRETINOIN (RETIN A)

Tretinoin has anecdotal support for use in the treatment of flat warts, but no controlled trials have demonstrated efficacy. Anecdotal experience suggests that tretinoin gel 0.01 to 0.025% applied daily to warts may speed their resolution. The drug may act by inducing inflammation or altering the differentiation state of the infected keratinocytes. The duration of therapy is not well characterized; however, a 3-month trial should provide ample opportunity to assess treatment success.

IMIQUIMOD (ALDARA)

Imiquimod is the first of a new generation of antiviral therapies that activate the host immune systems for wart eradication. Imiquimod is applied three times per week for 1 to 3 months until warts have been removed. This agent is indicated for genital warts but may have some efficacy on nongenital warts. As with podophyllitoxin, response rates for genital warts are as high as 70 percent for women but are on the order of 30 percent for men. In general, this agent works far better on mucous membrane warts than on dry skin warts. Patients experience side effects of burning, stinging, and pain. Imiquimod is likely to have some efficacy in the treatment of nongenital warts, but the response rates are not known. To increase efficacy in treating nongenital warts, occlusion or the concurrent use of keratolytics (to increase penetration) may be helpful.

CANTHARIDIN

Cantharidin consists of an extract of the blister beetle. This agent was previously available and widely used in the United States, but it is not currently approved by the U.S. Food and Drug Administration. This agent now must be imported without legal approval from Canada or other countries. Careful topical application of this solution induces impressive blister formation. The advantage of this approach is that it is often painless and can be an effective treatment for warts in children. It is also beneficial in treating plantar warts. It can cause severe blister reactions and may cause severe burning symptoms in occasional patients.

Oral Therapy

There are no demonstrated effective oral treatments for warts.

CIMETIDINE (TAGAMET)

Cimetidine was suggested as an "immune system enhancer" that was hypothesized to aid immunorejection of the wart virus. However, a placebo-controlled, double-blind trial showed that cimetidine is equal to placebo in efficacy in the treatment of common warts. Without a single convincing controlled trial, the value of cimetidine for warts remains dubious. However, it is a drug that is relatively free of side effects when used for short periods. Accordingly, many clinicians continue to advocate its use. The placebo effect may be helpful in treating warts; another factor may be that it gives anxious parents something to do for the wart until spontaneous resolution occurs. Thus, prolonged trials (3 to 6 months) should be considered. The usual dose is 30 to 40 mg/kg per day in three divided doses.

Intralesional Therapy

BLEOMYCIN

The cytostatic drug bleomycin has been used for verrucae that have failed to respond to other therapeutic modalities. Injection causes significant pain in the site. The use of this chemotherapeutic agent usually is limited by the expense and the possibility of extensive tissue necrosis in treated areas. Additionally, Raynaud's phenomenon has been reported to occur after injection into the fingertips.

Success rates with bleomycin are not well characterized. Both the success rate and the adverse event rate are probably highly operator-dependent. This treatment is probably best left to a few referral centers.

INTERFERON α

Interferon α is a cytokine that is used for the treatment of refractory warts. Expense, influenza-like side effects, and the frequency of required administration may limit its use. Furthermore, in a placebo-controlled trial using 1 or 3 million IU of interferon α2a administered subcutaneously three times weekly for 10 weeks in combination with ablative surgery, it was found that interferon in combination with ablative therapy is not significantly superior to placebo and ablative therapy in the treatment of anogenital warts.

Immunotherapeutic Agents

DIPHENCYPRONE

The induction of delayed-type hypersensitivity has been introduced for resistant viral warts. The possible advantage of this technique is that it is less painful and less destructive than most other modalities. No controlled trials have been performed, but an uncontrolled trial appears promising.

SQUARIC ACID DIBUTYLESTER

Squaric acid dibutylester (SADBE), a topical allergen, has been investigated in the treatment of patients with warts. Patients are sensitized with 2% SADBE in acetone, and then the warts are treated with a 0.1 or 0.01% SADBE application once a week or every other week. In an uncontrolled trial, about two-thirds of the patients had a good response. The main side effect is contact dermatitis.

Surgical Therapy

CRYOSURGERY

Ablation of warts with liquid nitrogen is a common and relatively effective treatment modality. This agent usually is applied to lesions for two 30-s freeze-thaw cycles. Crusting or blister formation may occur in treated areas, but scarring is rare. More than one treatment may be required for complete resolution of the warts. Pain associated with liquid nitrogen therapy limits its use in younger patients. Special precautions must be employed in darkly pigmented patients, who are more likely to have permanent depigmentmentation of the frozen skin. A potential complication is the development of a "ring" wart surrounding the treatment area.

A number of different liquid nitrogen application methods can be used, none with demonstrated superiority over the others. Spray applications are rapid and convenient. When cotton swabs are used to apply the nitrogen, one should remember that liquid nitrogen is an excellent cryopreservative for viruses. Accordingly, swabs should never be reused on other patients, and repetitive dipping of swabs into reservoirs is a potential source of nosocomial infection.

ELECTRODESICCATION AND/OR CURETTAGE

Electrodesiccation with or without curettage is another ablative therapy. Curettage may be performed without anesthesia, but electrodesiccation requires local anesthesia. As with excision (described below), there is a significant potential for secondary scarring with this procedure.

EXCISION AND/OR CURETTAGE

Surgical excision is limited to use in therapy for large, treatment-resistant warts because several less expensive, less aggressive therapies are available. Superficial curettage may be helpful for debulking large warts, especially on the feet.

CARBON DIOXIDE LASER

The carbon dioxide (CO_2) laser can be used to treat resistant warts but has some potential for scarring. Local anesthesia is required. The development of high peak power, short-pulse, or rapidly scanned resurfacing CO_2 lasers has significantly improved the safety and efficacy of using the CO_2 laser. Many lesions amenable to CO_2 laser vaporization can be treated with other, far less expensive treatment modalities, however, and it is the laser surgeon's responsibility to use the CO_2 laser only in cases in which it is demonstrably the best treatment option. A surgeon performing CO_2 laser ablation of HPV types that cause genital warts should be aware that these types have a predilection for producing upper airway mucosal warts. Accordingly, appropriate caution and plume removal techniques are important.

PULSED-DYE AND OTHER LASER SYSTEMS

The pulsed-dye laser targets the blood supply of the wart for destruction. It is a less painful laser treatment and has less potential for scarring than does the CO_2 laser. However, the pulsed-dye laser may not be as effective. Newer laser systems such as the Er:YAG laser with its extremely small zone of thermal damage may play a role in the treatment of warts.

Bibliography

Armstrong DK, Maw RD, Dinsmore WW, et al: Combined therapy trial with interferon alpha-2a and ablative therapy in the treatment of anogenital warts. *Genitour Med* 72:103, 1996.

Benton C: The management of viral warts. *Prac* 232:933, 1988.

Cobb MW: Human papillomavirus infection. *J Am Acad Dermatol* 22:547, 1990.

Edwards L, Ferenczy A, Eron L, et al: *Arch Dermatol* 134:25, 1998.

Gloster HM Jr, Roenigk RK: Risk of acquiring human papillomavirus from the plume produced by the carbon dioxide laser in the treatment of warts. *J Am Acad Dermatol* 32:436, 1995.

Hruza GJ: Laser treatment of warts and other epidermal and dermal lesions. *Dermatol Clin* 15:487, 1997.

Iijima S, Otsuka F: Contact immunotherapy with squaric acid dibutylester for warts. *Dermatology* 187:115, 1993.

Kainz JT, Kozel G, Haidvogl M, Smolle J: Homoeopathic versus placebo therapy of children with warts on the hands: A randomized, double-blind clinical trial. *Dermatology* 193:318, 1996.

Kimble-Haas S: Primary care treatment approach to nongenital verruca. *Nurse Pract* 21:29, 1996.

Landow K: Nongenital warts: When is treatment warranted? *Postgrad Med* 99:245, 1996.

Landsman MJ, Mancuso JE, Abramow SP: Diagnosis, pathophysiology, and treatment of plantar verruca. *Clin Podiatr Med Surg* 13:55, 1996.

Leigh IM, Glover MT: Cutaneous warts and tumours in immunosuppressed patients. *J R Soc Med* 88:61, 1995.

Luchtefeld MA: Perianal condylomata acuminata. *Surg Clin North Am* 74:1327, 1994.

Ordoukhanian E, Lane AT: Warts and molluscum contagiosum: Beware of treatments worse than the disease. *Postgrad Med* 101:223, 1997.

Rampen FH, Steijlen PM: Diphencyprone in the management of refractory palmoplantar and periungual warts: An open study. *Dermatology* 193:236, 1996.

Siegfried EC: Warts on children: An approach to therapy. *Pediatr Ann* 25:79, 1996.

Strand A, Brinkeborn RM, Siboulet A: Topical treatment of genital warts in men: An open study of podophyllotoxin cream compared with solution. *Genitour Med* 71:387, 1995.

Van der Velden EM, Ijsselmuiden OE, Drost BH, Baruchin AM: Dermatography with bleomycin as a new treatment for verrucae vulgaris. *Int J Dermatol* 36:145, 1997.

Von Krogh G: Clinical relevance and evaluation of genitoanal papilloma virus infection in the male. *Semin Dermatol* 11:229, 1992.

Wikstrom A, Hedblad MA, Johansson B, et al: The acetic acid test in evaluation of subclinical genital papillomavirus infection: A comparative study on penoscopy, histopathology, virology and scanning electron microscopy findings. *Genitour Med* 68:90, 1992.

Yilmaz E, Alpsoy E, Basaran E: Cimetidine therapy for warts: A placebo-controlled, double-blind study. *J Am Acad Dermatol* 34:1005, 1996.

Part 3

Skin Growths and Tumors

Epidermoid Cysts and Lipomas

Background   **Evaluation**
Etiology   **Treatment**
Clinical Presentation

Background

Cysts lined by squamous epithelium account for the majority of all cutaneous cysts that are encountered. Epidermoid cysts, which often are given the misnomer *sebaceous cysts,* are common benign neoplasms of follicular origin. Milia, which are smaller papular lesions that occur most frequently on the face, resemble tiny epidermoid cysts histologically. Inflammatory "cysts" in acne vulgaris are not true cysts; they are inflammatory nodules that lack a squamous epithelium and resolve spontaneously when the follicular and/or perifollicular inflammation resolves. Acne scarring can, however, give rise to permanent, noninflammatory epidermoid cysts. Lipomas are benign neoplasms that resemble normal adipose tissue both grossly and microscopically.

Etiology

Epidermoid cysts arise from the infundibular portion of the pilosebaceous unit (Fig. 14-1). The names used for this type of cyst include epidermal, epidermoid,

193

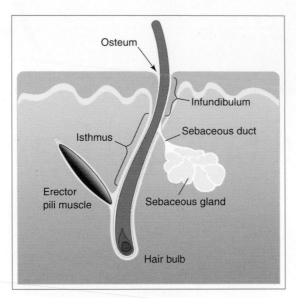

Figure 14-1

Origins of follicular cysts. The infundibulum of the hair follicle refers to the portion of the hair follicle between the ostium and the sebaceous duct. The lining of epidermoid cysts is thought to arise from the infundibular portion of the hair follicle. On this basis, these cysts also are called infundibular follicular cysts or follicular cysts, infundibular-type. Trichilemmal cysts (isthmus catagen cysts) are thought to arise from the isthmus of the hair follicle, the portion between the sebaceous duct and the insertion of the erector pili muscle.

epidermal inclusion, follicular infundibular, and keratin cysts. The walls of epidermoid cysts are made up of stratified squamous epithelium. Trichilemmal cysts are encountered second most frequently. Trichilemmal cysts have a clinical appearance similar to that of cysts of the follicular infundibulum, but occur on the scalp and arise from cells similar to those in the isthmus of the hair follicle (see Fig. 14-1). Thus, this cyst also is called an isthmus catagen or pilar cyst.

Epidermoid cysts may result from cutaneous injury from trauma or acne vulgaris. The vast majority arise without any evident trauma. There may be a hereditary tendency to develop these cysts. Multiple trichilemmal cysts seem to be inherited in an autosomal dominant fashion. Although clinicians have called epidermoid cysts *sebaceous cysts,* they have no sebaceous elements. There are true sebaceous cysts that are rarely encountered, with sebaceous elements in the walls. These lesions are more appropriately called steatocystoma simplex.

Lipomas are benign neoplasms of normal fat tissue. Typical locations include the trunk and extremities. On pathologic examination, the fat lobules appear larger than normal fat lobules and the normal architecture of the lobules is lost. An autosomal dominant familial form of lipomas, multiple familial lipomatosis, produces hundreds of lipomas in affected individuals. Benign symmetric lipomatosis (Madelung's disease) and adiposa dolorosa (Dercum's disease) are rare inherited multiple lipoma syndromes. Several variants of lipomas exist, including angiolipomas, hibernomas, and spindle cell and pleomorphic lipomas.

Clinical Presentation

Epidermoid cysts present as fluctuant, tense subcutaneous nodules that are freely movable and usually are found on the face, neck, trunk, and genitalia (Fig. 14-2). Their sizes range from 2 mm to several centimeters in diameter. A central punctum may or may not be recognized. If one is present, patients may report occasional drainage of foul-smelling keratin debris (Fig. 14-3). When these cysts occur on the genitalia, calcification is common. Trichilemmal cysts occur on the scalp, do not have a central punctum, and tend to be more smooth in appearance (Fig. 14-4). They also tend to calcify. Milia tend to occur on the face and may be single or multiple (Fig. 14-5). Secondary milia occur as a consequence of healing after trauma to the epidermis. When a cyst ruptures and its contents leak into the dermis, an intense foreign body reaction develops that results in pain, edema, erythema, drainage, and uncommonly secondary infection. In fact, inflamed and noninflamed cysts have nearly identical bacterial flora, suggesting that bacteria play little if any role in the pathogenesis of the inflammatory condition. After inflammation, the subsequent scarring may fix the cyst in place, with resultant fibrosis. Lipomas are soft, compressible subcutaneous nodules that range in size from a few

Figure 14-2

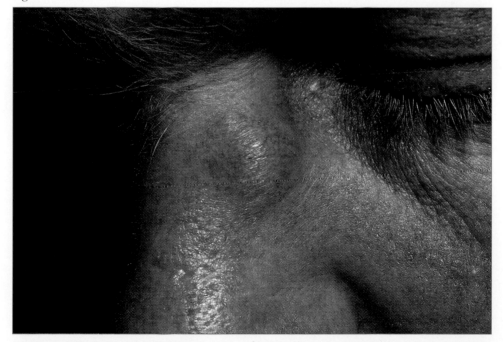

A typical epidermoid cyst of the face.

Figure 14-3

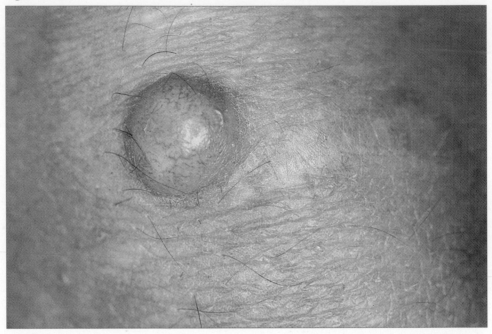

Epidermoid cysts have a central punctum and may drain a cheeselike material. (From Fitzpatrick TB et al: *Color Atlas and Synopsis of Clinical Dermatology, 3/e*. New York: McGraw-Hill, 1995, p. 164.)

millimeters to several centimeters in diameter. They are generally larger than epidermal cysts and occur mainly on the trunk, neck, and forearm. Lipomas are generally painful when compressed. The rubbery feel, the symmetric shape, and the unchanging character are the characteristics on which the diagnosis is made.

Evaluation

The diagnosis of epidermoid cysts, trichilemmal cysts, milia, and lipomas is almost always a clinical one that is based on the clinical findings discussed above. Further investigation is rarely warranted unless the appearance is atypical. When multiple epidermoid cysts occur in association with lipomas, fibromas, osteomas, and leiomyomas, the diagnosis of Gardner's syndrome should be considered. Patients with this autosomal dominant inherited disorder have polyposis of the colon and rectum in which malignant degeneration is common. When a subcutaneous nodule occurs on the scalp of a child, imaging of the area with x-ray, computed tomography (CT), or magnetic resonance imaging (MRI) should be undertaken before a planned excision to rule out an underlying meningocele.

Figure 14-4

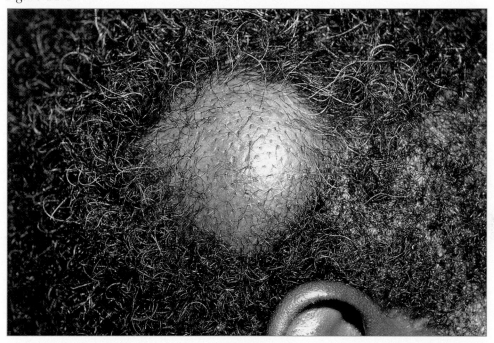

A tricholemmal cyst of the scalp. Trichilemmal cysts generally do not exhibit a central punctum. The overlying skin is smooth, and the cyst feels firm.

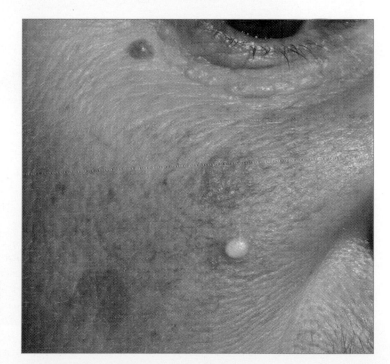

Figure 14-5

Milia are small (<0.3 cm) epidermoid cysts. They are common on the face and also can occur in scars or other sites of trauma. (From Fitzpatrick TB et al: *Color Atlas and Synopsis of Clinical Dermatology, 3/e*. New York: McGraw-Hill, 1995, p. 165.)

While liposarcomas are rare, any growing lipoma that reaches a size greater than 10 cm may require that a biopsy procedure be performed. Lipomas that occur in the midline of the back may suggest an underlying spinal abnormality, and clinicians should strongly consider radiographic procedures before any surgical intervention.

Treatment

Epidermoid cysts, trichilemmal cysts, milia, and lipomas are benign neoplasms that do not require treatment in most cases. However, patients may desire removal of these lesions for cosmetic or symptomatic reasons. The definitive treatment of epidermoid and trichilemmal cysts is removal of the cyst contents and wall. If one incises a cyst and removes the contents but does not remove the epithelial wall, the cyst will recur.

If patients desire removal, the cyst may be surgically removed using local anesthesia (Figs. 14-6 through 14-8). Cysts that have never been inflamed may be excised quickly and easily. Previously inflamed cysts with extensive scarring may be

Figure 14-6

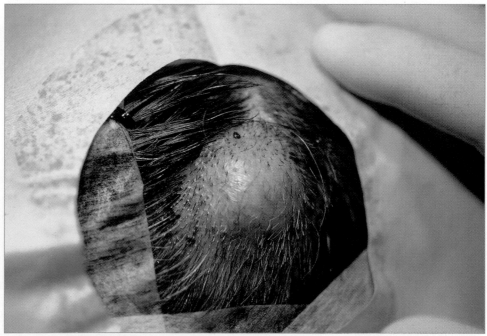

Preoperative preparation of a trichilemmal cyst of the scalp. The site is prepared by immobilizing or removing hairs that may interfere with the procedure. Local anesthesia is used.

Figure 14-7

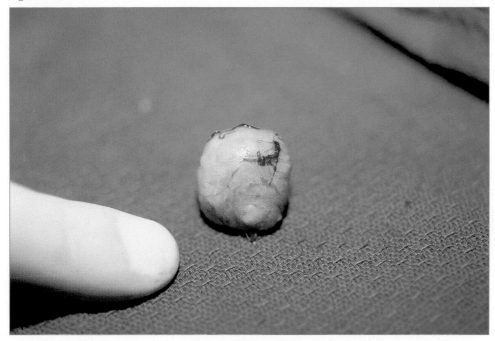

The cyst immediately after removal. To prevent recurrences, the entire cyst wall should be removed. This is best accomplished by removing the entire cyst without disturbing the cyst wall. To accomplish this, a small fusiform excision is made over the cyst to include the central punctum if it can be identified. Dissection is performed around the cyst, and then the cyst is delivered through the incision.

extraordinarily difficult to remove. Before anesthesia, delineating the surgical excision site and the extent of the cyst may help, as anesthesia tends to obscure the margins. If the cyst cannot be removed fully intact (see Fig. 14-7), removal of any residual cyst lining may be achieved by means of curettage with a dermal curette.

Trichilemmal cysts tend to "shell out" more easily than do epidermoid cysts. While care can be taken to dissect out the cyst wall without rupturing it, the fastest procedure entails enucleating the cyst (and its wall) through a small incision.

Inflamed cysts generally should not be surgically excised or enucleated. The resulting surgical scar will be large in comparison with the scar that will result from conservative treatment and excision after 1 to 3 months. Inflamed cysts may respond to intralesional corticosteroid injection or incision and drainage. Despite the widespread use of systemic antibiotic agents for inflamed cysts, there is no evidence that these antibiotics are helpful.

Milia can be treated by nicking the surface with a surgical blade and removing the contents with forceps, the blade, or a comedo extractor. Milia extraction can be performed with or without anesthesia, depending on the location of the site and the pain tolerance of the patient.

Lipomas require no surgical intervention. If the patient requests surgery, excision or liposuction generally is used. A small incision usually allows complete

Figure 14-8

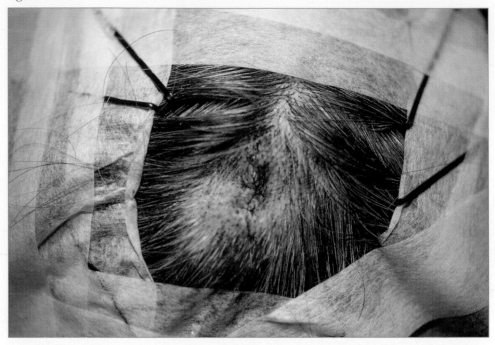

Sutured wound after cyst excision. The surgical wound of a cyst excision may be closed primary. A pressure dressing may be applied afterward for hemostasis, preventing filling of the remaining cavity with blood.

removal of fatty tissue, although it can be difficult to differentiate a lipoma from normal surrounding fat. Liposuction removes fat by sucking fatty tissue through a cannula with negative pressure applied. A smaller incision usually is created in the removal of lipomas by liposuction, but this is a time-consuming and more expensive procedure. The complications associated with liposuction include hematoma and seroma development.

Bibliography

Baldwin HE, Berck CM, Lynfield YL: Subcutaneous nodules of the scalp: Preoperative management. *J Am Acad Dermatol* 25:819, 1991.

Beacham BE: Common skin tumors of the elderly. *Am Fam Phys* 46:163, 1992.

Marshall KA, Kuhlmann TP, Horowitz JH, et al: Excision of multiple epidermal facial cysts in Gardner's syndrome. *Am J Surg* 150:615, 1985.

Narisawa Y, Kohda H: Cutaneous cysts of Gardner's syndrome are similar to follicular stem cells. *J Cutan Pathol* 22:115, 1995.

Nishimura M, Kohda H, Urabe A: Steatocystoma multiplex: A facial papular variant. *Arch Dermatol* 122:205, 1986.

Scott MA: Benign cutaneous neoplasms. *Prim Care Clin Office Prac* 16(4):643, 1989.

Melanoma

Background	***Prognosis***
Subtypes	***Treatment***
Etiology	Excision
Prevention	Lymph Node Dissection
Clinical Presentation	Other Treatments
Evaluation	***Summary***

Background

In the United States, the incidence of melanoma has almost tripled in the last 40 years and is increasing at a faster rate than that of any other cancer. It is estimated that by the year 2000, the lifetime risk will be 1 in 75. For a physician, the importance of recognizing melanoma lays in the high cure rate when melanoma is detected early and the dismal prognosis when it is discovered late.

Subtypes

Based on clinical and histologic characteristics, melanoma is classically divided into four types: superficial spreading melanoma, nodular melanoma, lentigo maligna melanoma, and acral lentiginous melanoma.

Superficial spreading melanoma (Figs. 15-1 through 15-4) accounts for about 70 percent of all melanomas. It usually presents in the fourth to fifth decade of life.

- difficult to Dx
brown colored

SSMs

Figure 15-1

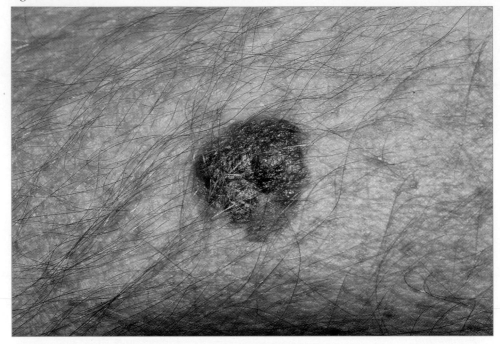

Malignant melanoma. The lesion is large and exhibits marked variation in color.

Figure 15-2

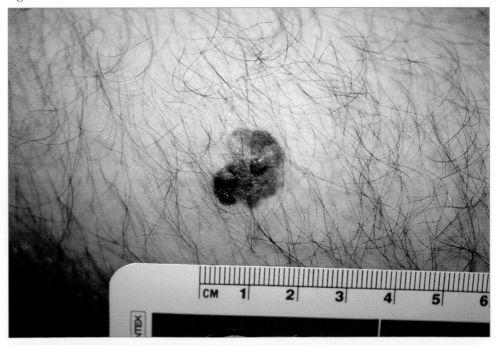

Malignant melanoma. This lesion has variation in color and a "notched" border.

Figure 15-3

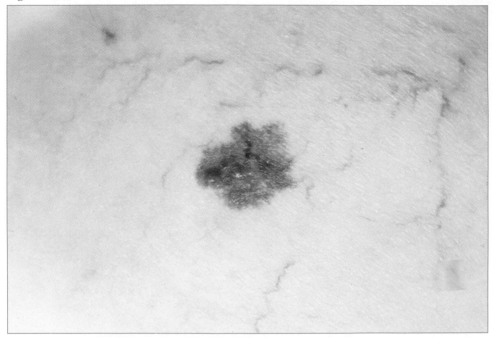

The borders of this melanoma are extremely irregular.

Figure 15-4

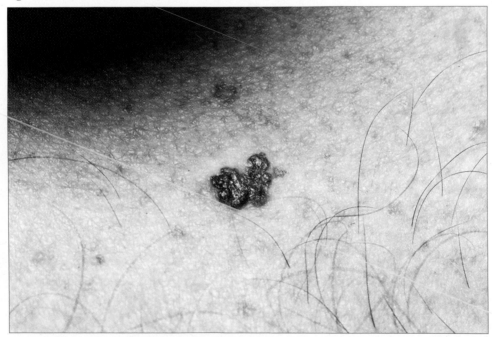

The asymmetry of the malignant melanoma is striking.

Figure 15-5

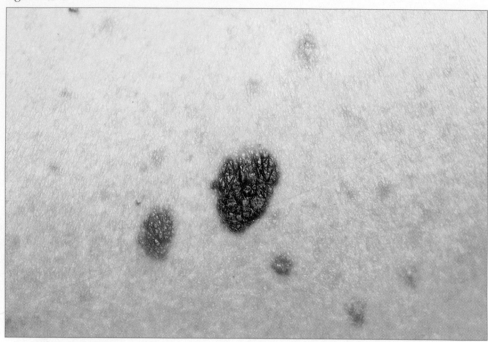

This melanoma has a more nodular appearance with less of a spreading character. The variation in color, asymmetry, and poorly defined border at one edge are features that indicate the need for removal.

Although superficial spreading melanoma may occur on any body surface, it is most commonly seen on the legs and back in women and on the back in men.

Nodular melanoma (Fig. 15-5) accounts for about 20 percent of melanomas. It occurs in a distribution similar to that of superficial spreading melanoma. Because nodular melanoma enters immediately into the vertical growth phase (see "Etiology," below), it is more likely to present as a rapidly growing pigmented papule or nodule.

Lentigo maligna melanoma (Fig. 15-6), which accounts for 5 percent of melanoma cases, arises from a precursor lesion known as lentigo maligna. Lentigo maligna is a form of melanoma in situ that occurs on sun-damaged skin. These lesions occur in the elderly on chronically sun-exposed areas such as the face, neck, and extensor forearms.

Acral lentiginous melanoma accounts for 2 to 10 percent of melanomas and is found on the palms, soles, and nail beds. This appears to be the only form of melanoma that is equally common in all races and is therefore the only form that is seen consistently in non-whites. It accounts for 35 to 90 percent of melanomas in African Americans, Asians, and Hispanics.

[Handwritten margin notes: easier to detect / looks like black bean on skin / in situ-hasnt invaded dermal/epidermal border / nail=hands & feet / chronically sun exposed areas]

Figure 15-6

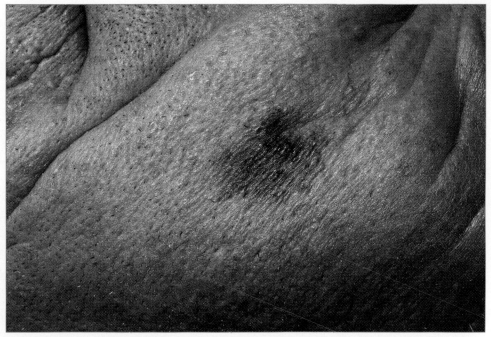

This melanoma has the features of lentigo meligna melanoma. This generally occurs on sun-damaged skin of the face. The lesion typically is thin, broad, and asymmetric with ill-defined borders.

melanoma → lighter skin, hair & eyes more common

Etiology

de novo = new

Cutaneous melanoma arises from the malignant transformation of melanocytes in the skin. It may arise de novo or from a precursor melanocytic nevus. Most studies suggest that only about one-third of melanomas develop from a precursor nevus. At the present time, the origin of the malignant transformation leading to a melanoma is unknown. Although a great deal of work has been done on the possible role of oncogenes and tumor suppressor genes in the development of melanoma, it does not seem that they play a major role in melanoma progression.

Once the malignant transformation has occurred, virtually all melanomas undergo a relatively long phase of radial growth during which the melanocytes spread centrifugally within the epidermis. The radial growth phase seems to lack metastatic potential. At some point the biological properties of the neoplastic cells change, and they enter the vertical growth stage with extension down into the dermis and eventually the subcutaneous fat. Cells in this phase are capable of metastasizing. The exception to this process is nodular melanoma, which has a very short or absent radial growth phase before beginning vertical growth.

Although the mechanism of the malignant transformation leading to malignant melanoma has not been found, multiple risk factors for the development of malignant melanoma have been noted. Total body nevus numbers appear to be strongly related to melanoma risk. In one study, the risk of melanoma rose 12-fold in those with more than 100 nevi compared with those with fewer than 10. Other risk factors include a prior history of melanoma, a personal history of melanoma, multiple large nevi, inability to tan, propensity to burn, freckling, proximity to the equator, and multiple atypical nevi. Additionally, an expanding body of literature supports the theory that the risk of melanoma depends in part on intense intermittent recreational sun exposure early in life.

A variety of melanoma syndromes have been described. In the atypical nevus syndrome, atypical melanocytic nevi occur in an individual with a family history of melanoma. These patients may have dozens of atypical nevi and have a lifetime risk for the development of melanoma that approaches 100 percent. Controversy arises, however, in the setting of nonfamilial or sporadic atypical nevi, which may occur in up to 10 percent of the general population. Although these individuals probably are at a higher risk for the development of melanoma, that risk is significantly lower than is the case in the familial type. Giant congenital nevi also represent a significant risk for the development of melanoma. The risk for melanoma developing in small or intermediate-size congenital nevi is not known but probably is small.

Prevention

It is not known whether melanoma can be prevented. Some melanoma, for instance, in the case of a familial syndrome, is hereditary and is not strictly preventable per se. However, some patients appear to have melanoma that is attributable, at least in part, to ultraviolet light and/or sun exposure. Because of the association of sunlight and melanoma and because of the effects of ultraviolet light in causing photoaging and nonmelanoma skin cancer, it is prudent to practice a comprehensive ultraviolet light exposure prevention program. This approach may include sunscreen, hats, and appropriate attire. Sunburn is not required for significant damage to occur; the majority of solar damage arises from repetitive suberythemogenic doses of ultraviolet irradiation.

These are straightforward and commonsense recommendations. The "controversy" regarding the effectiveness of sunscreen in the prevention of melanoma or the role of ultraviolet light in causing melanoma is vacuous and a distraction to the important message of ultraviolet protection. All forms of ultraviolet light (UVA, UVB, and UVC) damage skin (the presence of a tan is indicative of damage having been done), reduce cutaneous immune function, and may play a role in melanoma development. It is unlikely that there will ever be a randomized trial

[handwritten margin note: over 80% of lifetime exposure to UV occurs before 18]

that definitively proves that ultraviolet light exposure causes melanoma. Nevertheless, there is sufficient epidemiologic data to implicate exposure as a cause of melanoma and support the broad use of judicious protection against excessive sun exposure to reduce the incidence of melanoma.

Clinical Presentation

The patient often reports a new pigmented lesion or mole that has grown or changed in color, size, or shape (Figs. 15-1 through 15-8). The "ugly duckling sign," that is, the appearance of a pigmented lesion that is different from all the other pigmented lesions on the patient, should raise clinical suspicion (Figs. 15-9 and 15-10). For most patients with a melanoma, the lesion is asymptomatic. Pain, if present, usually is associated with a late presentation. Additional information, such as a personal or family history of melanoma, may raise the clinician's level of suspicion, but the key to the diagnosis lies in an examination of the lesion.

Figure 15-7

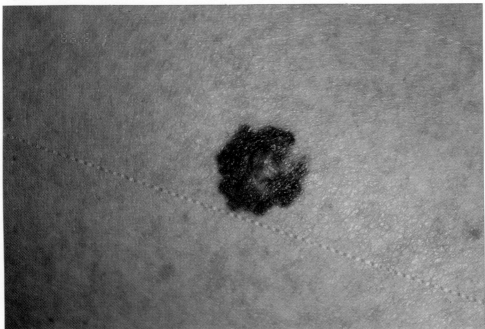

This melanoma exhibits irregular color and notched borders.

Figure 15-8

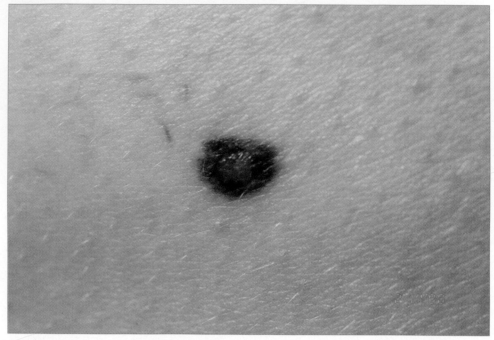

This lesion appears suspicious because of asymmetry and slightly irregular pigmentation. Biopsy revealed melanoma.

Figure 15-9

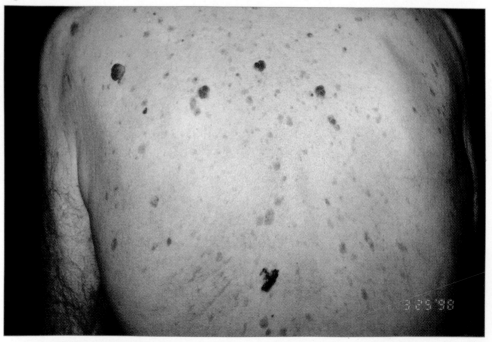

The "ugly duckling sign." The appearance of the pigmented lesion of the central, lower back is different from all the other pigmented lesions in this patient.

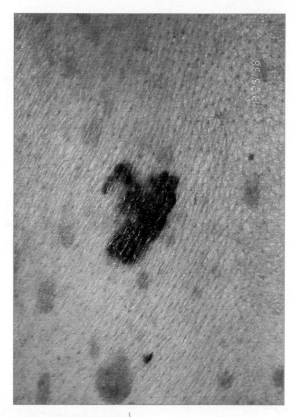

Figure 15-10

The "ugly duckling sign." A close-up view of the lesion in Fig. 15-9 reveals the large size, asymmetry, and irregular boders of a melanoma.

E=enlargement

The acronym ABCD is a useful reminder of some of the clinical features that should raise suspicion of melanoma in a pigmented lesion: *a*symmetry of the lesion, *b*order irregularity, *c*olor variegation or dark black color, and *d*iameter greater than 6 mm (the size of a pencil eraser). *highly suspicious*

The asymmetry of the lesion is the least useful criterion, but the other three criteria seem to have diagnostic significance. Additionally, the new appearance of papules, nodules, or ulceration in a pigmented lesion should prompt a great deal of suspicion. Another worrisome finding is regression in a pigmented lesion, which will appear as a new flat gray or white area in a previously completely pigmented lesion.

Large irregular pigmented lesions on the palms or soles should arouse suspicion of acral lentiginous melanoma. Small, symmetric, evenly pigmented lesions of the plam or sole are likely to be benign, but any change in these lesions indicates the need for biopsy. The subungual form of acral lentiginous melanoma may present only as a longitudinal pigmented band in the nail matrix. Although this may represent a relatively common condition seen in Black patients that is known as melanonychia striata, certain features should push one toward doing a biopsy. In particular, a single, new, or widening dark black band should raise

color is most important → color varies

Tyndale effect - grows horizontal then grows vertical → color changes due to depth of lesion

melanoma esp. if affects proximal nail fold → indicates malignancy - not painful

suspicion. Hutchinson's sign, in which pigmentation spreads onto the proximal nail fold is indicative of melanoma.

Lentigo maligna or lentigo maligna melanoma will presents as an irregularly bordered patch on sun-damaged skin, particularly the face, of elderly patients. It usually has been present for years and demonstrates multiple shades of brown and black, often with other areas of hypopigmentation.

If the diagnosis of melanoma is suspected, a careful examination of regional lymph nodes should be performed before a biopsy of the lesion is done. This is the case because the biopsy may lead to regional lymphadenopathy, which could be a confounding factor in later examinations and staging of the patient.

A pigmented lesion should be examined carefully to exclude the possibility that it represents a seborrheic keratosis. Seborrheic keratoses may be irregularly colored and may have irregular borders. However, they typically have a "stuck-on" waxy appearance with a scaling, pebbly surface (Figs. 15-11 and 15-12). Atypical nevi may appear very similar to melanoma (Fig. 15-13) and require a biopsy for accurate diagnosis.

could be confused w/ nodular melanoma ↓ blacker & smoother

Figure 15-11

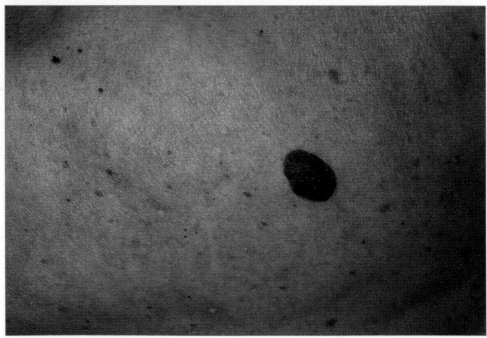

Seborrheic keratoses are characterized by a waxy, "stuck-on" appearance.

Figure 15-12

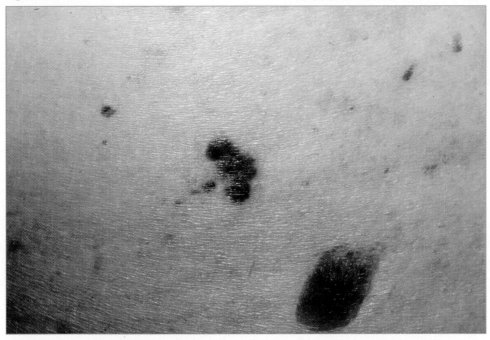

Seborrheic keratoses may mimic melanoma. This seborrheic keratosis is asymmetric and has notched borders. Biopsy or referral is indicated when the diagnosis is not clear.

Figure 15-13

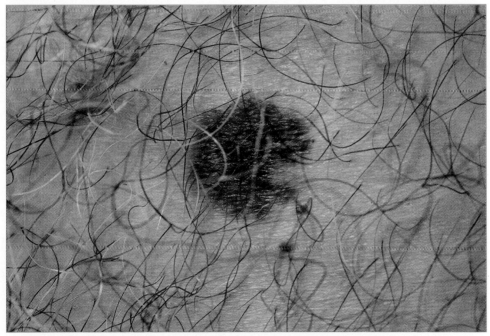

Atypical nevus. This nevus has features of melanoma, including irregular pigmentation and an irregular notched border. Biopsy of such a lesion is necessary to exclude the possibility of melanoma.

Evaluation

When a suspicious lesion has been identified (as discussed above), the clinician should perform a biopsy or refer the patient. This decision should be based on the clinician's comfort with and expertise in the differential diagnosis of benign from malignant skin lesions (that is, the sensitivity and specificity for identifying melanoma), skill at performing the biopsy procedure, and facility in interpreting the resulting histologic diagnosis of the pigmented lesion. Each of these three components offers complexities. If it is unclear to the clinician whether a biopsy is needed, the clinician does not have the expertise to obtain an appropriate biopsy specimen, or the clinician has difficulty interpreting the diagnosis offered by the pathologist, a referral probably is indicated.

When the decision to biopsy has been made, the entire lesion should be removed in the procedure so that the pathologist can identify the features that distinguish a benign process from a malignant process. The entire lesion must be removed because the important features include the character of the proliferation at the deep and lateral margins. Different biopsy techniques may be used (shave, punch, or excision) as long as the biopsy specimen contains the lateral and deep aspects of the tumor. Biopsy techniques that do not remove the entire lesion should be considered only if the lesion is so large that complete excision would require a flap or graft to repair, or if the lesion is in a cosmetically important site, such as the face, where full excision would lead to an unacceptable cosmetic outcome if the lesion was found to be benign.

There is no evidence that incomplete removal adversely affects the patient's prognosis, but it could affect the ability to render accurate prognostic information. If a shave procedure is done that is not of sufficient depth, prognostic information may be lost, but the procedure itself will have no effect on the prognosis of the patient.

One would expect that the histologic interpretation of pigmented lesions would be straightforward (benign versus malignant); unfortunately, it is not. In many cases, pathologists have a level of uncertainty in making a definitive diagnosis. The resulting interpretations fall into a benign, malignant, and some variation of "I don't know" classification scheme. To complicate matters, the terminology used by different pathologists is such that a term that means "benign" to one pathologist may mean "I don't know" or even "malignant" to another.

Certain ambiguous terms commonly appear in pathology reports of pigmented lesions. The clinician must communicate with the pathologist to understand how the pathologist uses terms that may indicate a benign process or a process with malignant potential:

Atypical nevus
Dysplastic nevus: variations include "mild," "moderate," and "severe" dysplasia
Atypical melanocytic proliferation

Juvenile melanoma
Nevus with unusual cytologic or architectural features

Histopathologic examination of melanocytic tumors is notoriously difficult, and great dermatopathologic experience helps. Clinicians who remove melanocytic lesions should read pathology reports carefully and consider discussing the findings with the pathologist. Biopsy reports from some pathologists may use older, misleading terminology such as *juvenile melanoma* instead of the newer term *Spitz nevus* (spindle and epithelioid nevus). These "juvenile melanomas" are benign. By contrast, a true melanoma in situ may be described as "dysplastic nevus with marked junctional activity" or an "atypical nevus," and a comment may describe characteristic malignant features. Failure to remove melanoma in situ completely may result in progression to invasive melanoma and death. True communication between the clinician and the pathologist is essential and in many cases must be supplemented by clinicopathologic correlation. If an extremely suspicious melanocytic lesion is interpreted by a general pathologist as being benign, the clinician should consider asking for a consultation. The reverse may be the case, with a benign melanocytic tumor being misinterpreted as malignant.

Once a patient has been diagnosed with melanoma, there is no standard of care for evaluation that every clinician would agree is appropriate. For patients with relatively thin melanomas (<1 mm), any tests beyond histopathologic evaluation of the biopsy specimen have little diagnostic value. That is, there is no proven value of chest radiography, blood chemistry or hematologic evaluation, and other testing. In patients with thick melanomas, clinicians should consider performing a chest x-ray and serum liver function tests.

Lymph node dissection techniques may be helpful in assessing the prognosis, but there is no convincing evidence that these invasive procedures affect the prognosis. The same may be said of more advanced techniques, such as the sentinel lymph node biopsy approach. Unless controlled trials demonstrate the clinical utility of these approaches in improving the prognosis, lymph node sampling is best considered a staging or diagnostic procedure rather than a therapeutic procedure. It is clear that patients who have lymph node metastases have a poorer prognosis than do those who have no metastases.

Prognosis

Once melanoma is diagnosed, assuming there that are no obvious nodal or distant metastases, the most important factor in deciding on the prognosis and treatment is the tumor thickness determined from the biopsy specimen. Melanoma in situ can be cured completely with surgical excision. Some melanomas are in situ in some locations but are deeper in other areas. Unless the complete tumor has

Table 15-1 *Deeper lesions, less likely to be curable*

Five-Year Survival Rates for Melanoma

Percent Surviving for 5 Years	Size, mm
100	0
95	≤0.74
85	0.75–1.4
66	1.50–3.9
46	≥4.0

been examined histologically, an accurate assessment of the true depth cannot be assigned. The 5-year survival rates for melanomas based on tumor thickness are shown in Table 15-1.

Additional histologic factors offer further prognostic information. For instance, microscopic evidence of regression, the briskness of the lymphocytic infiltrate, and the number of mitoses per high-power field may all provide further information on the risk of metastasis. This type of histopathologic information is generally available from the pathology report or from a discussion with the pathologist. As might be expected, patients with lymph node involvement have a significantly poorer prognosis than do those with lesions of similar thickness but no involvement of nodes. Patients with multiple sites of distant metastases are generally incurable and have a median survival of 6 months.

Patients can never be correctly told that their disease has been cured. There have been reports of recurrence of melanoma after 35 years of freedom from disease. Of course, as each disease-free year goes by, the risk of recurrence decreases. Providing optimism and support for patients over the long term is a more reasonable strategy than using the term *cure*.

Treatment

Excision

Initial management consists primarily of surgical excision of the melanoma (Table 15-2). Even if the initial excisional biopsy seemed to remove the entire lesion, it is recommended that reexcision be performed if adequate margins were not obtained. The current recommendations for surgical margins are dependent on tumor thickness. No study to date has demonstrated the clinical utility of wide margin excision. For instance, when 1-cm excision margins were compared with 3-cm margins, there was no prognostic difference in any subset of patients. The same is true of 2-cm margins compared with 4- or 5-cm margins. Nevertheless, a reasonable

Table 15-2

Algorithm for the Treatment of Melanoma

> Remove the primary lesion in its entirety
>   Surgical margins are based on thickness:
>   In situ lesions: 0.5 cm
>   Melanoma ≤1mm: 1 cm
>   Melanoma 1–4 mm: 1–3 cm
>   Melanoma >4 mm: 3 cm
>   Consider micrographic surgery in cosmetically critical areas
> Lymph node dissection
>   Palpable nodes: recommend lymph node dissection
>   No palpable nodes: lymph node dissection controversial
>   Not needed for melanoma <1 mm or >4 mm
>   Debatable for melanoma >1 mm and <4mm
> Adjunctive therapy
>   Interferon α: increases survival in patients with regional lymph node involvement
>   Palliative chemotherapy, radiation, excision of metastases
>   Immunotherapy not of proven benefit
> Long-term follow-up
>   History and physical; consider chest x-ray and liver function tests

recommendation is that in situ lesions have excision performed with a 0.5-cm margin of clinically normal skin and a layer of subcutaneous fat. Melanoma ≤1 mm in thickness should be excised with a 1.0-cm margin of clinically normal skin down to the deep fascia. Melanoma 1 to 4 mm in thickness should be excised with 1- to 3-cm margins down to the fascia. Melanoma >4 mm in thickness should be excised with 3-cm margins down to the fascia. For patients with melanoma involving cosmetically critical areas such as the face, Mohs micrographic surgery may be a tissue-sparing therapeutic option.

Lymph Node Dissection   *enlarged, rubbery, non-tender*

Patients with palpable lymph nodes should undergo lymph node dissection for prognostic purposes and to decrease the tumor burden. For patients without evidence of lymph node involvement, there is controversy about whether they should undergo elective lymph node dissection. At present, controlled trials have not demonstrated therapeutic efficacy of elective lymph node dissection. However, some clinicians argue that lymph node dissection may offer prognostic information and influence the use of adjuvant therapy. It generally is agreed that for patients with thin lesions (<1.0 mm), the risk of regional lymph node metastases is so small that it does not justify the morbidity associated with elective lymph node dissection. Conversely, for patients with thick (>4.0 mm) melanomas, the probability that the melanoma has already spread beyond the regional lymph nodes is so high that the procedure is not likely to confer therapeutic benefit. However, for patients with melanomas of intermediate thickness (>1 mm but <4 mm), the debate continues about the potential benefits of this procedure.

Other Treatments

At present, the only officially recognized adjuvant therapy for patients without evidence of distant metastases is interferon α. It has thus far only been shown to increase survival in the subset of patients with regional lymph node involvement. This agent does not appear to offer a cure; instead, it represents a palliative intervention.

In widespread metastatic melanoma, the goal of therapy should be palliation, as this condition generally is incurable. Chemotherapy, radiation, surgical excision of solitary metastases, and interferon have all been employed with marginal success.

There is no convincing evidence that immunotherapy offers benefit over placebo. A randomized, controlled trial of 761 subjects receiving adjuvant chemotherapy, immunotherapy, or immunochemotherapy was performed by the World Health Organization International Melanoma Group. Subjects with stage II cutaneous melanoma anywhere on the body or with pathologic stage I melanoma of the trunk were subjected to wide local excision and excisional regional lymphadenectomy, and the results were compared with those of surgery plus chemotherapy with dacarbazine, surgery plus immunotherapy with bacille Calmette-Guerin vaccine, and surgery plus chemotherapy combined with immunotherapy. No prognostic difference could be demonstrated between any of the study groups. Until controlled trial results demonstrate benefit from such immunotherapy, one must conclude that this approach has little value.

For patients without evidence of widespread disease at presentation, long-term follow-up is an important aspect of management. These patients should be monitored for melanoma recurrence and metastasis. Additionally, patients who have had a previous melanoma are at reasonable risk of developing additional melanomas. The most sensitive tool for detecting recurrences and metastases remains a thorough history and physical examination. In the absence of clinical evidence of metastatic disease, for patients with melanomas >0.75 mm in thickness, yearly chest x-ray and liver function tests should be considered, although their cost efficacy has never been evaluated.

Summary

Primary care clinicians are in an excellent position to identify melanomas in an early and curable phase. Removing early melanomas is one of the indisputable lifesaving procedures clinicians can perform. The acronym ABCD is a useful reminder of the clinical features that should raise suspicion of melanoma in a pigmented lesion: *a*symmetry of the lesion, *b*order irregularity, *c*olor variegation or dark black color, and *d*iameter greater than 6 mm.

Bibliography

Brown M: Staging and prognosis of melanoma. *Sem Cutan Med Surg* 16:113, 1997.

Cohen LM: Lentigo maligna and lentigo maligna melanoma. *J Am Acad Dermatol* 35:1016, 1996.

Greenstein DS, Rogers GS: Management of stage I malignant melanoma. *Dermatol Surg* 22:730, 1996.

Huth JF: Surgical treatment of malignant melanoma. *Semin Cutan Med Surg* 16:159, 1997.

Liu T, Soong S: Epidemiology of malignant melanoma. *Surg Clin North Am* 76:1205, 1996.

McGovern TW, Litaker MS: Clinical predictors of malignant pigmented lesions: A comparison of the Glasgow seven-point checklist and the American Cancer Society's ABCDs of pigmented lesions. *J Dermatol Surg Oncol* 18:22, 1992.

Penneys NS: Excision of melanoma after initial biopsy: An immunohistochemical study. *J Am Acad Dermatol* 13:995, 1985.

Perez IR, Fenske NA, Brozena SJ. Malignant melanoma: Differential diagnosis of the pigmented lesion. *Sem Surg Oncol* 9:168, 1993.

Ringborg U, Andersson R, Eldh J, et al: Resection margins of 2 versus 5 cm for cutaneous malignant melanoma with a tumor thickness of 0.8 to 2.0 mm: Randomized study by the Swedish Melanoma Study Group. *Cancer* 77:1809, 1996.

Tahery DP, Moy RL: Recurrent malignant melanoma following a 35-year disease-free interval. *J Dermatol Surg Oncol* 19:161, 1993.

Veronesi U, Adamus J, Aubert C, et al: A randomized trial of adjuvant chemotherapy and immunotherapy in cutaneous melanoma. *New Engl J Med* 307:913, 1982.

Veronesi U, Adamus J, Bandiera DC, et al: Inefficacy of immediate node dissection in stage 1 melanoma of the limbs. *New Engl J Med* 297:627, 1977.

Veronesi U, Adamus J, Bandiera DC, et al: Stage I melanoma of the limbs: Immediate versus delayed node dissection. *Tumori* 66:373, 1980.

Veronesi U, Cascinelli N, Adamus J, et al: Thin stage I primary cutaneous malignant melanoma: Comparison of excision with margins of 1 or 3 cm. *New Engl J Med* 318:1159, 1988.

Chapter 16

Melanocytic Nevi

Background	***Evaluation***
Etiology	***Treatment***
Clinical Presentation	

Background

Melanocytic nevi are abnormal but benign proliferations of melanocytes in the skin that histologically demonstrate the formation of "nests" of cells. As defined by Harple (1995), "Nevi are visible, circumscribed, long-lasting lesions of the skin or the neighboring mucosa, reflecting genetic mosaicism." These lesions may be present at birth, in which case they are referred to as congenital melanocytic nevi, or may appear at any time after birth, most commonly in childhood, in which case they are called acquired melanocytic nevi.

Congenital melanocytic nevi are present in approximately 1 percent of all newborns. These lesions have been arbitrarily subdivided on the basis of size into small (less than 1.5 cm), intermediate (1.5 to 19.9 cm), and giant (20 cm and larger). Giant congenital melanocytic nevi are found approximately 200 times less frequently than are small ones. The importance of giant congenital melanocytic nevi lies in their potential for transformation to melanoma, with a reported lifetime risk of 5 to 15 percent.

Acquired melanocytic nevi begin to appear after the first 6 to 12 months of life and increase in number until the second or third decade, after which they begin to regress. Acquired melanocytic nevi may be categorized on the basis of the histologic location of the melanocytes into junctional nevi (melanocytes in epidermis), compound nevi (melanocytes in epidermis and dermis), and intradermal nevi (melanocytes in dermis). A variation on these types are "halo nevi," in which there is inflammation that causes destruction of the nevus.

Etiology

All melanocytic nevi, both congenital and acquired, are composed of nevus cells that probably are derived from neural crest melanoblasts or their progeny. Nevus cells are simply melanocytes that have accumulated in larger than normal aggregations. These cells tend to aggregate in nests in the epidermis and/or dermis, with congenital melanocytic nevi tending to have their cells extend deeper into the dermis.

The number and size of melanocytic nevi in an individual probably are determined by a combination of genetic and environmental factors. The prevalence of acquired melanocytic nevi is substantially higher in whites than in blacks and Asians. Nevus counts are generally higher in those with light skin color and a propensity to burn in the sun. It is likely that excessive solar exposure, particularly in childhood, increases the prevalence of melanocytic nevi.

The other significance of atypical nevi lies their presence in the atypical nevus syndrome. Originally described in 1978, this syndrome involves kindreds with individuals having multiple atypical-appearing nevi and a markedly increased risk of melanoma. These patients, who have many highly atypical nevi and a strong family history of melanoma in first-degree relatives (mother, father, sibling, or children), may have a lifetime risk of melanoma that approaches 100 percent. However, the sporadic subtype, in which patients have multiple atypical nevi but no family history of melanoma, has only a slight increase in melanoma risk. While it is common for patients to have a "dysplastic nevus" (conferring little if any risk for melanoma), it is rare for patients to have the "dysplastic nevus syndrome" (in which there are numerous dysplastic nevi, a strong family history of melanoma, and a high risk for the development of melanoma).

Clinical Presentation

Congenital melanocytic nevi are generally asymptomatic. A history of the nevus initially having been noted at or shortly after birth is valuable, since clinically these lesions may be indistinguishable from acquired melanocytic nevi. Congenital melanocytic nevi tend to be larger than acquired melanocytic nevi, but there is tremendous variability in the size of the individual lesions (Figs. 16-1 and 16-2). The most common locations for congenital melanocytic nevi are the trunk and

Figure 16-1

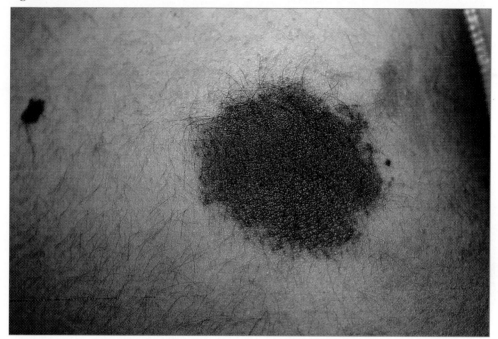

Congenital nevi of intermediate size.

Figure 16-2

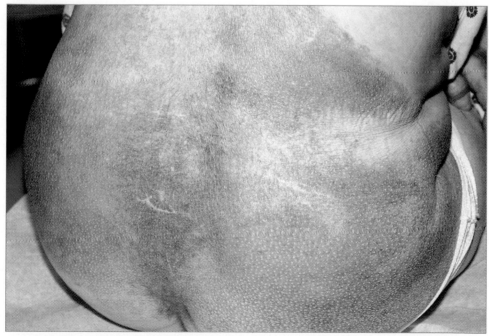

Large congenital melanocytic nevus in an adult.

thighs, although they may be located on any cutaneous surface. Congenital melanocytic nevi are usually well marginated, are round or oval, and distort skin surface markings. They tend to be only minimally elevated at birth, although the surface appearance may be anything form smooth to verrucous to lobular. Pigmentation tends to be a uniform medium brown to dark brown. Dark terminal hairs may be present at birth or appear later. During childhood, congenital melanocytic nevi may become darker and more papular and develop increased numbers of dark terminal hairs, with an acceleration of this phenomenon during puberty.

Any history of a significant change in the appearance of the lesions, particularly in giant congenital melanocytic nevi, should prompt concern regarding possible malignant transformation of the congenital melanocytic nevi to melanoma. In patients with giant or multiple congenital melanocytic nevi of the posterior axial area, head, or neck, there is a significant frequency of neurocutaneous melanosis. Neurocutaneous melanosis is defined as the presence of the nevi described above in addition to leptomeningeal melanocytosis. Clues to the presence of neurocutaneous melanosis include seizures, mental retardation, and focal neurologic deficits and signs of increased intracranial pressure.

Acquired melanocytic nevi are usually asymptomatic, and these patients are most likely to present with concerns regarding either the cosmetic appearance of the lesions or the possibility that they represent melanoma. However, occasionally, acquired melanocytic nevi that have a significant papular component may become irritated by local frictional processes. Acquired melanocytic nevi typically range from 1 mm to 1 cm in diameter, have a round to oval shape, and have relatively demarcated smooth borders.

Both congenital and acquired nevi can be categorized as follows.

Junctional nevi are flat or minimally raised macules ranging in color from light brown to black. Minimal or no distortion of skin surface markings is noted, and the nevus is not palpable. The nevi appear as dark freckles (Fig. 16-3A).

Compound nevi are obviously raised to visual inspection and palpation. They are often papillomatous and range in color from light tan to brownish black (Fig. 16-3B).

Intradermal nevi are also papular with a smooth or papillary surface. They may be skin-colored to light brown and tend to have a rubbery texture to palpation (Fig. 16-3C).

Halo nevi are nevi that have been depigmented as a result of a normal immunologic response. The halo refers to a depigmented patch surrounding the normal nevus (Fig. 16-4). If the nevus in the center of the halo is normal-appearing, these nevi are usually benign.

Atypical (dysplastic) nevi are the most challenging melanocytic nevus for the physician. These nevi clinically demonstrate variegated colors of tan, brown, black, and pink with irregular outlines and a diameter generally from 5 to 15 mm. They are found predominantly on the torso and the proximal upper extremities. Single or multiple lesions may be found on a single patient (Fig. 16-5).

These lesions are important for two reasons. First, they may be difficult to differentiate from melanoma. As their clinical description indicates, atypical nevi may

Figure 16-3

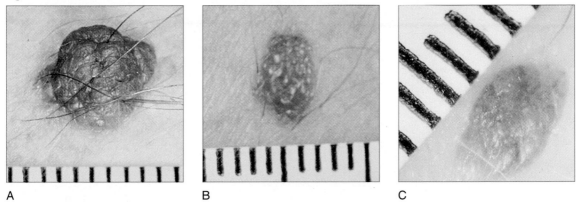

A   B   C

Nevi. *A.* The junctional nevus is a flat, dark symmetric macule with sharp distinct borders. *B.* The compound nevus has features both of a dermal nevus (a raised palpable papule) and of a junctional nevus (hyperpigmentation). *C.* The dermal nevus is a flesh-colored symmetric papule. (From Freedberg I et al, eds: *Dermatology in General Medicine, 5/e.* New York, McGraw-Hill, 1999, p. 101.)

Figure 16-4

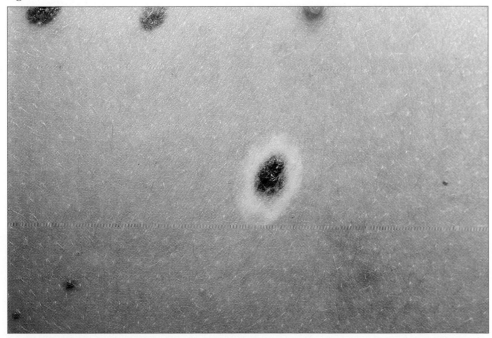

A typical halo nevus.

Figure 16-5

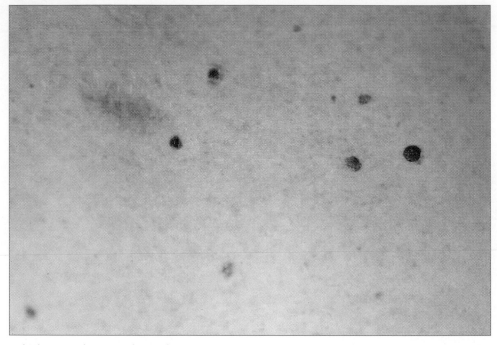

Multiple atypical nevi on the trunk.

simulate many of the clinical characteristics of melanoma. Patients' risk for the development of melanoma is related to the number of both typical and atypical nevi, and large numbers of clinically atypical nevi raise the lifetime melanoma risk substantially.

The second significance of atypical nevi lies in their presence in the atypical nevus syndrome, as was discussed above. Patients with many highly atypical nevi and a strong family history of melanoma in first-degree relatives (mother, father, sibling, or children) may have a lifetime risk of melanoma that approaches 100 percent. More commonly, however, a patient may have multiple atypical nevi and no family history of melanoma; in this case, there is only a slight increase in melanoma risk. The most common scenario is a patient who has only one or two "dysplastic" nevi; this by itself does not portend a high risk of melanoma.

Evaluation

For lesions suspected of being melanoma, clinicians should consider a shave or excisional biopsy or refer the patient for further evaluation (Chap. 15). The clinical differentiation between an atypical nevus and a melanoma may not always be made on clinical grounds. There has been recent interest in the dermatoscope, a hand-held magnifying tool for careful visual analysis of atypical nevi. Unfortunately, there is no clear evidence that this instrument is more sensitive or specific for differentiating melanocytic lesions than careful unmagnified examination. Nevertheless, some clinicians strongly recommend dermatoscopy.

The biopsy procedure produces scarring. In certain locations, such as the upper chest and back in younger patients, this scarring is unavoidable. The clinician and patient together should weigh the advantages of histologic sampling and early melanoma discovery with potential cure against the scarring potential.

Treatment

Most acquired melanocytic nevi require no treatment. Patients may ask for the removal of acquired melanocytic nevi that are cosmetically undesirable or are subject to constant irritation. When benign nevi are removed in this fashion, this is purely a cosmetic procedure.

However, clinicians should strongly consider performing a biopsy or refer the patient for evaluation if the lesion appears clinically atypical. Features that may indicate the need for removal include variation in the color of the nevus, asymmetry, poorly defined borders, and any change that has been noted by the patient. Another helpful sign is the "ugly duckling" sign, which refers to a nevus that appears different from all the others. Because of the high mortality of melanoma and the low morbidity of skin biopsy procedures, a low threshold for performing a biopsy of a suspicious lesion is indicated.

The goal of the biopsy is to obtain enough tissue for the pathologist to identify the features needed to distinguish a benign process from a malignant process. These features include the character of the lesion at its deep and lateral margins. Different biopsy techniques may be used (shave, punch, or excision) as long as the biopsy specimen contains the lateral and deep aspects of the tumor.

Patients who have been diagnosed as having large numbers of atypical nevi, particularly those with a family history of melanoma (atypical nevus syndrome), require careful follow-up. The ideal follow-up regimen has not been well characterized. These patients should be followed routinely at 4- to 12-month intervals (the shorter interval would be used in a patient who has had melanoma or has numerous dysplastic nevi plus a strong family history of melanoma). Occasionally clinicians advocate serial photography to monitor the large number of atypical lesions.

Giant congenital melanocytic nevi require early evaluation for surgical removal because the greatest risk of malignant degeneration exists before age 10 years. Surgery usually is postponed until the infant is 10 to 14 months of age or older, when the risk of anesthesia does not outweigh the potential for future melanoma.

The excision may be total or staged and may require the use of tissue expanders and skin grafts. When the size or site of a giant congenital melanocytic nevi precludes its surgical excision, there is a need for diligent lifetime follow-up with a low threshold for punch or incisional biopsies of suspicious-appearing areas within the nevus. Surgical excision does not remove all the melanocytes in the nevus; it merely represents an aggressive debulking procedure. Benign melanocytes may be found in the underlying muscle and may "metastasize" to lymph nodes.

The management of small and intermediate-size congenital melanocytic nevi is controversial. Although excision of these lesions is easier than it is for giant congenital melanocytic nevi, their potential for transformation into melanoma is unclear. There is no clear evidence that small or intermediate-size congenital melanocytic nevi have a greater malignant transformation risk than in normal skin. Despite this absence of a clear benefit, some clinicians have advocated removal of intermediate sized congenital melanocytic nevi when patients are old enough to tolerate local anesthesia. It is highly likely that the risk of death from general anesthesia exceeds the risk of melanoma death. The decision to excise these lesions can be delayed until the child is approximately 10 years old, as the risk of melanoma in this setting is rare before age 12. At present, it is reasonable to inform each patient of the potential risk of melanoma, although this risk is small and controversial. The patient and his or her guardian may then decide whether they wish to have the lesion excised or monitor it for suspicious changes.

Dermabrasion and Q-switched ruby laser therapy have been suggested for the removal of congenital melanocytic nevi. Although a more acceptable cosmetic result may be achieved, these modalities do not remove as many of the melanocytes as does excision. Accordingly, one could postulate without scientific evidence that the risk of malignant transformation may be higher with superficial ablative procedures than it is with excisional surgery.

Bibliography

Chamlin SL, Williams ML: Moles and melanoma. *Curr Opin Pediatr* 10:398, 1998.

Gallagher RP, McLean DI: The epidemiology of acquired melanocytic nevi. *Dermatol Clin* 13:595, 1995.

Grulich AE, Bataille V, Swerdlow AJ, et al: Naevi and pigmentary characteristics as risk factors for melanoma in a high-risk population: A case-control study in New South Wales, Australia. *Intern J Cancer* 67:485, 1996.

Happle R: What is a nevus? A proposed definition of a common medical term. *Dermatology* 191:1, 1995.

Harth Y, Friedman-Birnbaum R, Linn S: Influence of cumulative sun exposure on the prevalence of common acquired nevi. *J Am Acad Dermatol* 27:21, 1992.

Magana-Garcia M, Ackerman AB: What are nevus cells? *Am J Dermatopathol* 12:93, 1990.

Mooi WJ: The dysplastic naevus. *J Clin Pathol* 50:711, 1997.

Roth ME, Grant-Kels JM: Important melanocytic lesions in childhood and adolescence. *Pediatr Clin North Am* 38:791, 1991.

Schleicher SM, Lim SJ: Congenital nevi. *Int J Dermatol* 34:825, 1995.

Seykora J, Elder D: Dysplastic nevi and other risk markers for melanoma. *Semin Oncol* 23:682, 1996.

Swerdlow AJ, English JS, Qiao Z: The risk of melanoma in patients with congenital nevi: A cohort study. *J Am Acad Dermatol* 32:595, 1995.

Tucker MA, Halpern A, Holly EA, et al: Clinically recognized dysplastic nevi: A central risk factor for cutaneous melanoma. *JAMA* 277:1439, 1997.

Weinstock MA, Goldstein MG, Dube CE, et al: Basic skin cancer triage for teaching melanoma detection. *J Am Acad Dermatol* 34:1063, 1996.

Premalignant and Malignant Nonmelanoma Skin Tumors

Background

Nonmelanoma precancerous and cancerous neoplasms are closely related to long-term solar exposure and the absence of adequate protective melanin for that amount of exposure. Actinic keratoses are the most common type of premalignant skin lesion. Basal cell carcinoma is the most common malignancy found in humans and is characterized by slow growth and an extremely small risk of metastasis. Squamous cell carcinoma is the second most common skin cancer and has a much lower rate of metastasis than does squamous cell carcinoma in noncutaneous areas.

Risk Factors

The primary risk factor for the development of actinic keratosis (AK), basal cell carcinoma (BCC), and squamous cell carcinoma (SCC) is cumulative exposure to ultraviolet light in susceptible individuals. Those at the highest risk are fair-skinned patients with light-colored eyes. Fair skin and light eye color imply smaller amounts of intracutaneous melanin. In high-latitude climates with little solar exposure, fair skin may enable people to produce adequate quantities of activated vitamin D and smaller intracutaneous melanin levels are not problematic because solar radiation is less at high latitudes. However, closer to the equator, pigmentation is required to shield the skin from excessive solar damage. The highest skin cancer rates are found in areas in which many people can trace ancestry to northern Europe and where solar exposure is abundant, such as Australia and the southern United States.

Other forms of ultraviolet radiation, such as phototherapy for conditions such as psoriasis, predispose patients to develop more AK, BCC, and SCC. Radiation-induced SCC or BCC usually develops from repeated doses of small amounts of radiation, such as with x-rays. Patients who have undergone allograft transplantation and similarly immunocompromised persons are at higher risk for the development of AK and SCC. Chronic scarring from conditions such as burns, chronic cutaneous lupus erythematosus, and ulcers also raises the risk for developing SCC in affected areas. Genital SCC occurs more frequently in uncircumcised men and patients with preexisting condyloma acuminata.

Behavior is also a risk factor, because it predicts sun exposure. Agricultural and horticultural workers, construction workers, lifeguards, and similarly exposed workers are at greatly increased risk. Similarly, golfers, boat owners, gardeners, sunbathers, and other outdoor leisure enthusiasts have a higher likelihood of developing skin cancer. Even a few months to a few years of intense solar exposure may increase the long-term risk of oncogenesis greatly.

The vast majority of nonmelanoma skin cancers are located on the face, neck, upper shoulders and upper neck, and posterior arms. These are the areas that receive the greatest lifetime cumulative doses of ultraviolet radiation. When one takes into account the amount of body surface area at different body sites, one finds that the risk of BCC is highest on the most sun-exposed face (ears, nose, and cheeks), lower on the less exposed face (forehead, eyebrow, chin, and jaw), and lower yet on the least exposed face (area within the orbit and nasolabial fold) (Raasch and associates 1998). This differs for SCC somewhat, and SCC incidence is higher on the less exposed face than it is on the higher exposed face and the sun-exposed upper limbs. Nonmelanoma skin cancers of both types occur on the trunk and elsewhere but are much less common there than on the face and arms.

Pathophysiology

Nonmelanoma skin cancers arise from epidermal squamous cells. AKs arise in the same cell type as SCCs, and the factor differentiating the two is the depth of dysplasia. AKs are on one end of the spectrum where dysplasia is found in the partial thickness of the epidermis, SCC in situ involves the entire thickness of the epidermis, and the dysplastic cells of invasive SCC are found extending into the dermis. AK has a small but definite potential to develop into SCC if left untreated. Although it is not possible to prove directly that chronic ultraviolet radiation causes skin cancer, the evidence supporting that idea is compelling. Precancerous and cancerous cutaneous lesions arise primarily on sun-exposed areas of the skin in patients who are more susceptible to the damaging effects of ultraviolet radiation. Tumor induction by ultraviolet radiation also depends on other factors, such as interactions with other tumor initiators and promoters. Immunologic factors such as tumor suppression by the host are important, as evidenced by the increased risk of skin cancers and precancerous lesions in immunosuppressed patients. The carcinogenic process probably involves multiple steps, beginning with induction that results in DNA damage and followed by the proliferation of cancerous cells.

Much less is known about the induction of BCC, since animal models are not well established. It is likely that some of the same mechanisms occur in other oncogenic models, including that for SCC.

Symptoms

AK begins most often as asymptomatic papules that can be palpated more easily than they can be seen. As the papules become more developed or more extensive, patients may become aware of these scaling lesions, which sometimes peel off and then recur. Hypertrophic AK can become ulcerated and bleed easily.

BCC and SCC usually grow slowly, and a patient may be unaware of the lesion for several months or years. These lesions may become ulcerated and bleed easily, and many patients describe them as "a sore that won't heal."

AK, BCC, and SCC can become tender, but it is sometimes the appearance of the lesions that prompts the patient to visit a physician. Some keratoacanthomas, a variant of SCC, grow rapidly and ulcerate over a period of weeks to months.

Physical Examination

Actinic Keratoses

Actinic keratoses are subtle and may appear as slightly erythematous to hyperpig-mented scaling macules and papules measuring 2 to 5 mm in diameter on sun-exposed areas, especially the face, ears, neck, and forearms and hands (Figs. 17-1 through 17-3). The more hypertrophic type of AK has a thick hyperkeratotic surface and a palpable but not markedly indurated base. Pigmented AK are usually slightly larger and have a definite brown to black color. Actinic cheilitis, a form of AK most often found on the lower lip, presents as hyperkeratosis with focal areas of leukoplakia.

Basal Cell Carcinoma

Basal cell carcinomas have multiple clinical variants, each with a somewhat unique presentation. Most appear on sun-exposed areas of the head and neck, trunk, and

Figure 17-1

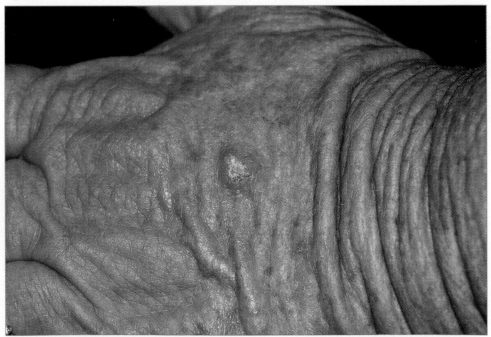

Actinic keratosis on the sun-exposed portion of the hand.

Figure 17-2

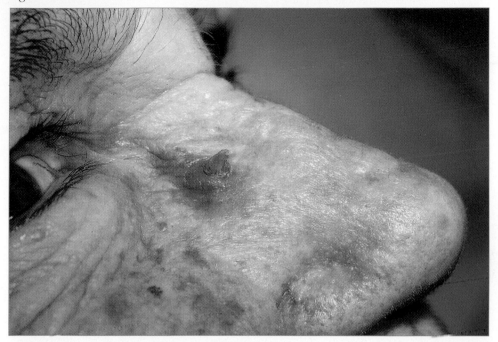

An actinic keratosis presenting as a cutaneous horn.

Figure 17-3

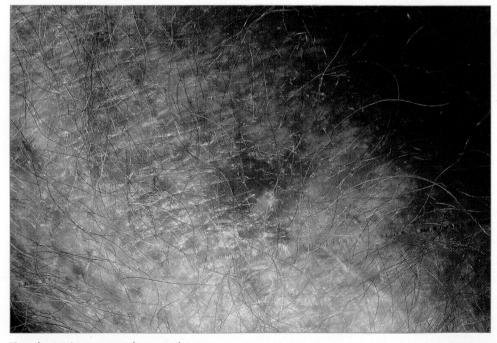

Hyperkeratotic cutaneous horn on the arm.

Figure 17-4

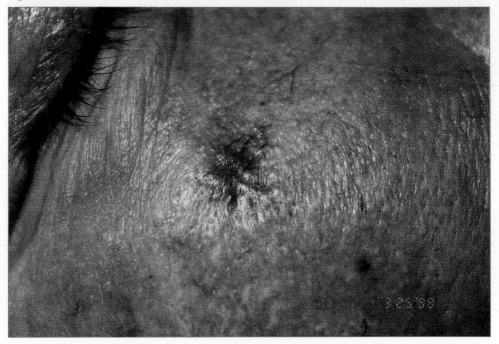

Typical nodular basal cell carcinomas.

extremities. The most common subtype, the nodular variant, presents as a pearly to erythematous papule that may have associated rolled borders and contain tiny telangiectasias (Figs. 17-4 through 17-7). Central ulceration may be present. Superficial BCCs are sharply marginated circular erythematous plaques that may have a subtle raised border (Fig. 17-8). Pigmented BCCs resemble either nodular or superficial BCC, but have a blue-black pigmentation, particularly pigment stippling in the periphery. Morpheaform BCC is an uncommon subtype that presents as an irregular, waxy, slightly elevated plaque resembling a scar. A fibroepithelioma of Pinkus is another uncommon subtype that presents as a sessile, flesh-colored papule on the trunk. All these subtypes vary greatly in size from barely perceptible to huge, ulcerating tumors that destroy normal anatomic structures.

Squamous Cell Carcinoma

Squamous cell carcinoma typically presents as an erythematous to flesh-colored hyperkeratotic plaque found in about the same anatomic distribution as BCC (Figs. 17-9 through 17-11). Ulceration may be associated with these lesions. Bowen's disease, a form of SCC in situ, is characterized by a well-circumscribed erythematous plaque with overlying hyperkeratosis. It has a predilection for developing on the trunk but may occur anywhere on sun-exposed skin. Erythroplasia of Queyrat is

Figure 17-5

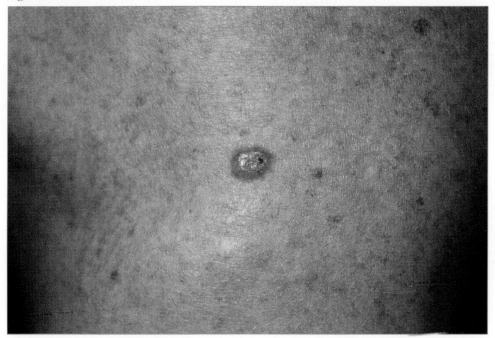

Typical nodular basal cell carcinomas.

Figure 17-6

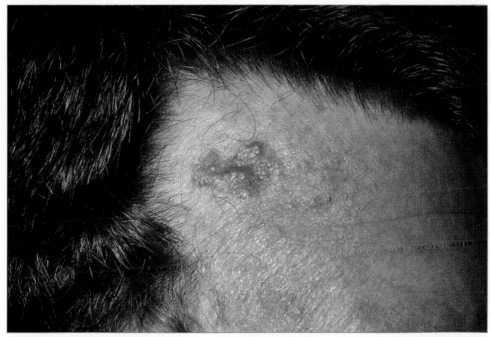

Typical nodular basal cell carcinomas.

Figure 17-7

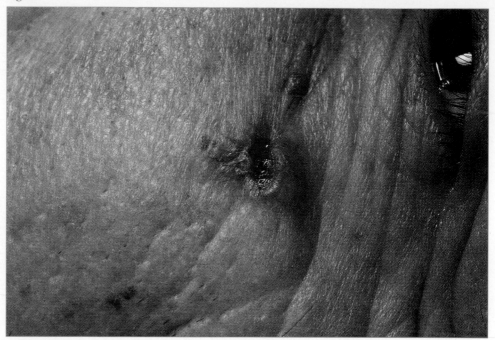

Typical nodular basal cell carcinomas.

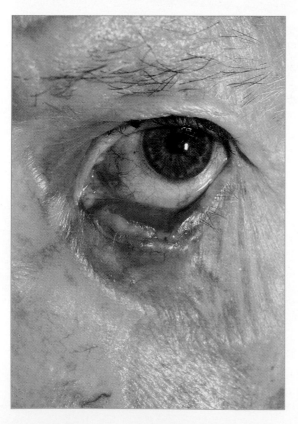

Figure 17-8

Superficial spreading basal cell carcinoma on the trunk.

Figure 17-9

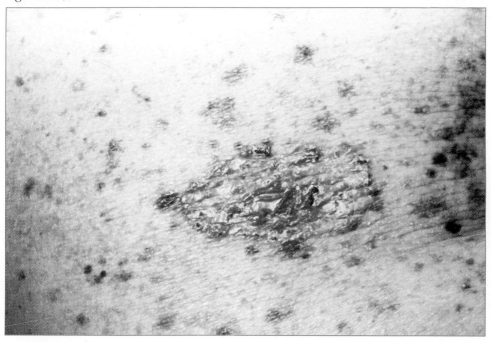

Squamous cell carcinomas arising on sun-exposed skin.

another form of SCC in situ that presents as brightly erythematous plaques on the glans penis or penile shaft (Fig. 17-12). Bowenoid papulosis is a human papillomavirus–associated SCC in situ that is characterized by tan to flesh-colored flat-topped papules on the external genitalia. Keratoacanthoma is a histologic variant of SCC that presents as a rapidly growing, crater-shaped, flesh-colored to erythematous nodule with a central keratinous plug on sun-exposed skin. The latter lesion is "benign" but has a tremendeous ability to cause local destruction. Keratoacanthomas as a rule do not metastasize. However, histologic distinction of SCC from keratoacanthomas is not always possible.

Evaluation

The diagnosis of AK, BCC, and SCC is a clinical diagnosis, and if confirmation is required, a skin biopsy must be performed. Lesions that are felt to be entirely consistent precancers or cancers may not require biopsy before treatment, depending on the comfort of the patient and physician with the diagnosis. The risk of failing to perform a diagnostic biopsy before definitive treatment is that the patient will

Figure 17-10

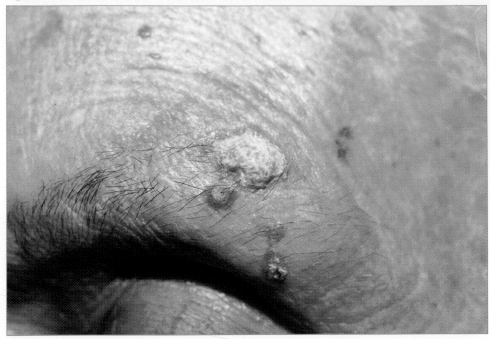

Squamous cell carcinomas arising on sun-exposed skin.

Figure 17-11

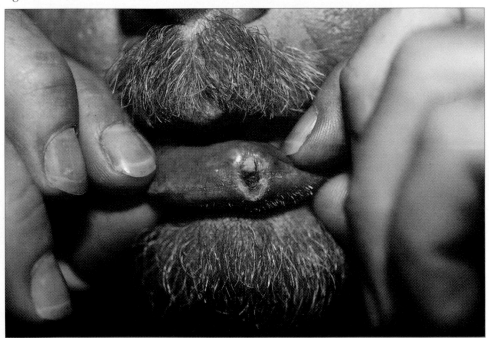

Squamous cell carcinomas arising on sun-exposed skin.

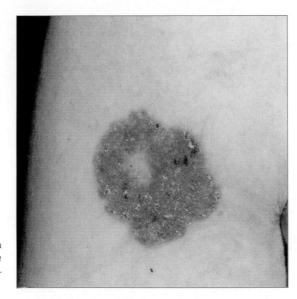

Figure 17-12

Squamous cell carcinoima in situ (From Freedberg I et al, eds.: *Dermatology in General Medicine, 5/e*. New York, Mc-Graw-Hill, 1999, p. 840.)

have considerably more scarring in the event of a misdiagnosis. The problem with performing a biopsy is that it subjects the patient to additional expense and an additional appointment is required if the lesion proves to be cancerous. Some clinicians always perform biopsy procedures before initiating definitive treatment on suspected lesions, while others perform biopsies on indeterminate lesions.

A biopsy strictly for diagnosis optimally consists of a shave biopsy of a small portion of the lesion. Punch biopsies are a less desirable choice, as they make subsequent electrodesiccation and curettage more difficult to perform. Excisional biopsies may be definitive if adequate margins are taken.

A lymph node examination should be considered with SCC on specific mucous membrane locations, such as the lip. It is reasonable to perform this examination on all patients, but the risk of non–mucous membrane SCC metastasis is low.

Complications

AK may evolve into SCC if left untreated. The presence of AK appears to be necessary for the development of SCC. Marks and colleagues (1998) mapped AKs and followed 1,689 people over a 5-year period. When accurate mapping of both SCCs and preexisting solar keratoses was available, it was found that 60 percent of SCCs arose from a lesion diagnosed clinically as an AK in the previous year. The risk of malignant transformation of an individual AK within 1 year was about 1 in 1,000. Accordingly, AKs are clearly premalignant, but the risk of any single lesion over a decade is modest.

BCC has an extremely low risk of metastasis. SCC of the skin also has a low metastatic risk, but this risk is raised when the carcinoma arises on a mucous membrane. Carcinomas are locally destructive if left untreated, and this destruction may compromise any nearby anatomic structure. In immunocompromised patients, the risk of metastasis is greatly increased.

Management

Photoprotection for All Premalignant and Malignant Neoplasms

The optimal approach in preventing the development of skin cancers and precancerous lesions is protection from excessive sun exposure. This entails applying sunscreen, wearing a hat and protective clothing, and avoiding direct sun exposure at the peak hours of 10 A.M. to 2 P.M. Sunscreen has been proved in controlled trials to decrease the numbers of AKs that develop. Accordingly, all high-risk patients should be counseled about solar protection techniques.

Actinic Keratoses

Actinic keratoses may be left untreated, but the patient and physician should understand that there is a small but measurable risk of progression to SCC. AK also may be treated with ablative therapies, including liquid nitrogen cryotherapy and curettage. Since cryosurgery causes erythema and occasional blistering, this procedure should not be performed within a week before an important business or social event. Care should be taken to avoid depigmenting the skin, as melanocytes are highly sensitive to cold injury. Depending on the depth of the lesion and the body site, individual lesions may require freezes ranging from 2 to 10 s. Also, numerous different techniques, ranging from disposable cotton swabs to dozens of cryosurgical devices (Fig. 17-13), are available, precluding a discussion of technique in this chapter. The technique is dependent on the equipment, the lesion, and the patient. After cryosurgery, we advise patients to wash the areas with conventional soap one to three times per day and apply an antibiotic ointment such as Polysporin to the area after cleansing.

Some clinicians use curettage instead of cryosurgery. There do not appear to be benefits of one approach over the other, and the results of both are highly operator-dependent.

Topical 5-fluorouracil (5-FU) can be used for extensive AK twice a day for 3 to 4 weeks. This approach is extremely useful in clearing large photodamaged areas. We generally advise patients to spread a thin layer of cream over the entire areas to be treated twice per day, taking care to wash their hands before touching their eyes. This approach induces erythema, crusting, and pain in treatment areas, and

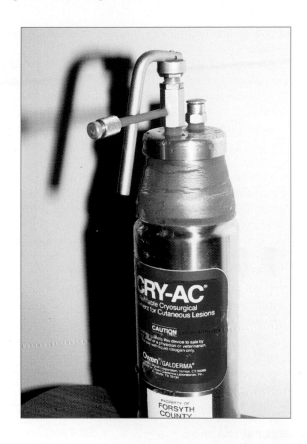

Figure 17-13

Example of a typical cryosurgical device.

the erythema may take 1 to 3 months to fade. We prefer to treat patients in the winter months to avoid medication-acquired photosensitivity and sweating into ulcerated skin. Before therapy, adequate counseling should be given by experienced physicians to make certain that patients understand this treatment modality and its side effects.

Basal Cell Carcinoma and Squamous Cell Carcinoma

OVERVIEW

The treatment of BCC or SCC depends on the size, location, and nature of the underlying tissue. For instance, excisional techniques may be more preferable on the face in patients with large numbers of wrinkles and even pigmentation, since the scar may be less obvious. Secondary considerations should include patient expectations, patient age, concomitant medications, and the methods employed in treating previous skin cancers in the patient. Medications are of key importance in the preoperative evaluation of patients. For instance, a patient being treated for unstable angina with aspirin and coumadin undoubtably will have significant bleeding during the removal procedure as well as the postoperative period. Thus, excisions are technically more difficult to accomplish than are destruction techniques.

All removal techniques should be accompanied by the submission of specimens for histopathologic confirmation. This is important in terms of verifying the type of tumor removed as well as making sure that certain patients are treated appropriately.

In a systematic review of published studies over a 40-year period on recurrence rates for primary BCC, 5-year recurrence rates were as follows: Mohs micrographic surgery, 1.0 percent; excision, 10.1 percent; electrodesiccation and curettage, 7.7 percent; radiation therapy, 8.7 percent; and cryosurgery, 7.5 percent. When tumors recur, clinicians should consider Mohs surgery, as the tumor pathology may be more infiltrating than it is for the average tumor. Recurrences also may be handled by reexcision or reablation if there is abundant tissue available for the removal process (e.g., on the chest) and if the tumor margins are distinct.

ELECTROCOAGULATION AND CURETTAGE

Tumor destruction by electrocoagulation in combination with curettage is a commonly used procedure for BCC and occasionally for SCC (Fig. 17-14). This procedure usually is reserved for tumors that are small (less than 1 cm in diameter),

Figure 17-14

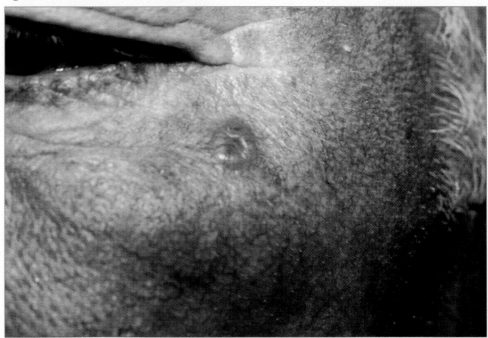

A

Removal of nodular basal cell carcinoma by electrodesiccation and curettage. *A.* Tumor. *B.* After tissue cleansing, local anesthesia is instilled to effect a ring block. *C.* Sharp curettage is performed vigorously until the operator can feel and see no residual tumor. *D.* Electrodesiccation is performed to the base and wound margin. *E.* The final appearance before dressing the wound.

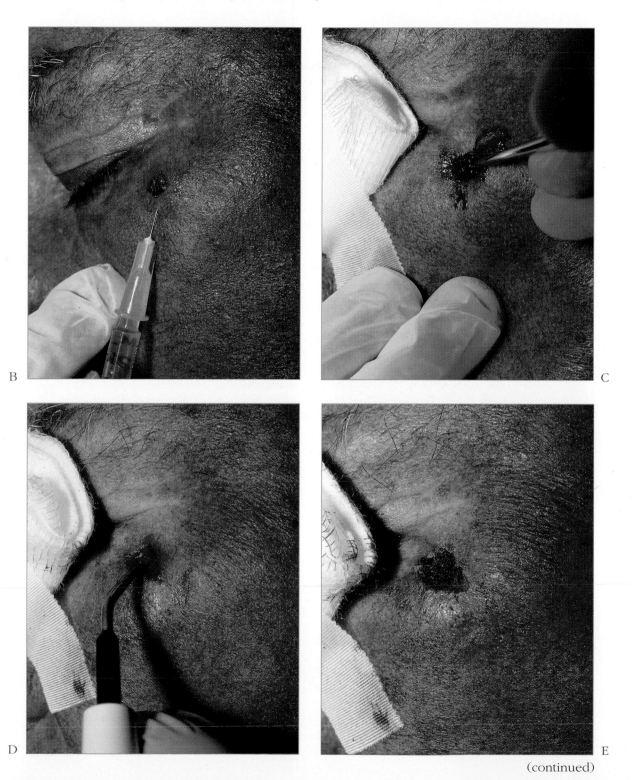

(continued)

have well-demarcated boundaries, occur in less cosmetically sensitive areas (e.g., the back or extremities), or occur on flat surfaces such as the forehead or cheek. The benefits of this procedure are that the procedure is quite effective, the scar is typically no larger than the original tumor, the procedure is relatively simple to perform for experienced clinicians, and the procedure usually can be performed despite ongoing treatment with anticoagulant medications. Disadvantages include an unnatural-appearing, depressed porcelein-white scar, and, as with excision, this procedure carries the risk of infection and nerve and blood vessel damage. This procedure may not be cosmetically optimal on faces that have an even skin tone in which a white patch would be cosmetically undesirable.

More skilled clinicians have better cure rates than do less skilled clinicians. Physicians who perform many procedures weekly have far better results than do those who perform this procedure on an occasional basis.

EXCISION

Surgical excision with 2- to 4-mm margins can be used to eradicate most BCCs and SCCs. The benefits of this procedure are that the procedure is quite effective and the scar is linear and thus often can be made to conform to natural lines of the face. The disadvantages include the fact that this procedure requires skilled technique, can be difficult in the setting of anticoagulant therapy, and carries the risk of nerve and blood vessel damage. As with electrocoagulation and curettage, more skilled clinicians achieve better cure rates than do less skilled clinicians. In our medical center, dermatologists have far higher histologic tumor clearance rates with surgical excision than do general, plastic, and otolaryngologic surgeons. This difference may be due in large part to experience and cannot be accounted for on the basis of tumor site, tumor size, tumor histology, patient's sex, or patient's age. Studies have shown that surgical outcomes for serious conditions are improved by increased surgical volumes, and the same appears to hold for "minor" surgical procedures.

MOHS MICROGRAPHIC SURGERY

Mohs is the only technique for treating cancer in which the clinician examines the actual tumor margins rather than examining a sampling of the margins. That is, pathologists evaluate the "margins" of traditional excision specimens by examining supposedly representative vertical sections obtained by "breadloafing" specimens. This approach examines a small portion of the actual surgical margins. By contrast, the Mohs technique involves the examination of 100 percent of the tumor margins.

As Dzubow (1994) has summarized, the strength of the Mohs procedure lies in the technique of sequential layered removal, precise tissue orientation and mapping, and the application of horizontally oriented frozen sections. Tumor excision is accomplished in staged small layers, and each removal stage is followed by a processing and mapping session.

The tissue that is removed is subdivided into small pieces, with each piece color-coded and oriented. A map is drawn to document the anatomic location of each specimen along with the pattern of the orienting dyes. The tissue is cut horizontally, resulting in a section that displays the entire perimeter and undersurface of that section. Barring processing inadequacies, errors in interpreting the microscopic sections, and noncontinuity (multifocality) of the tumor, the cure rate for local control of nonmelanoma skin cancer is virtually 100 percent.

After examination of the Mohs microscopic sections, the previously drawn map is marked to indicate areas containing residual tumor. The patient returns to the operating suite, and another layer is excised in the precise site of tumor presence. Accordingly, removal of surrounding healthy tissue is minimized. The operating-processing cycle continues until all of the tumor is removed. After histologic tumor clearance, immediate reconstruction is often possible.

Typical carcinomas that can be considered for Mohs micrographic excision include recurrent carcinomas, carcinomas arising in a scar, ill-defined or larger carcinomas, and those in areas in need of maximal tissue conservation (nose, ear, eyelids, lip, fingers, toes). The Mohs technique uses fresh tissue to gain microscopic control of tumor removal and is performed by specially trained surgeons. The advantages of this technique are that it has the highest cure rate of any approach and has the best cosmetic outcome of any technique. The disadvantages include the fact that it is time-consuming for patients and physicians and as a result is quite costly. In relative cost terms, it is no more expensive than performing a simple excision in an outpatient surgical center when operating room time and equipment are billed.

RADIATION

Radiation therapy is a consideration for patients who have inoperable skin cancers. These tumors may be so large that they involve half the patient's face and the surgical options are sometimes undesirable. The cosmetic outcomes are not always good, particularly a decade after removal. Treatment typically consists of 2 or more weeks of daily radiation doses. The advantages are that it is nonoperative and can eradicate deep tumors. The disadvantages include poor long-term cosmetic outcome, high cost, difficult treatment schedules, and complex subsequent surgery.

CRYOTHERAPY

Cryotherapy has a few vocal supporters, but it is a less commonly performed technique because of perioperative morbidity in treating BCC and SCC. Cryosurgery, like other deep, destructive techniques for skin cancer, requires local anesthesia. Cryotherapy is much more uncomfortable for patients postoperatively than are other destructive procedures, such as electrodesiccation and curettage. Accordingly, cryotherapy should be used only by physicians experienced in this procedure; none of the authors of this chapter employ this approach.

CHEMOTHERAPY

Interferon α has been used in the treatment of nonmelanoma skin cancer. Unfortunately, cure rates are inferior to those obtained by surgical removal or ablation, and expense and toxicity are significant barriers. Accordingly, this approach is unlikely to gain favor.

Prognosis

Careful follow-up is crucial for patients diagnosed with an AK, BCC, or SCC. These patients should be seen at least once yearly. Patients who have over 10 AKs or have a history of multiple SCC or BCC probably should be seen two to four times per year. Patients with any of these premalignant or malignant skin neoplasms are at greatly increased risk of developing other premalignant or malignant skin neoplasms. Early detection and removal of premalignant lesions and malignant skin cancers improves the cosmetic outcome and function and may decrease the overall cost of care.

Bibliography

Dzubow LM: Mohs surgery. Lancet 343(8895):433, 1994.

Epstein JH: Nonmelanoma skin cancer. *Comp Ther* 22:179, 1996.

Fleming ID, Amonette R, Monaghan T, et al: Principles of management of basal and squamous cell carcinoma of the skin. *Cancer* 75(Suppl 2):699, 1995.

Goldberg DP: Assessment and surgical treatment of basal cell skin cancer. *Clin Plast Surg* 24:673, 1997.

Lang PG: Variables to consider in the management of nonmelanoma skin cancer. *J Geriatr Dermatol* 4:231, 1996.

Marks R, Motley RJ: Skin cancer: Recognition and treatment. *Drugs* 50:48, 1995.

Marks R, Rennie G, Selwood T: The relationship of basal cell carcinomas and squamous cell carcinomas to solar keratoses. *Arch Dermatol* 124:1039, 1988.

Marks R, Rennie G, Selwood TS: Malignant transformation of solar keratoses to squamous cell carcinoma. *Lancet* 1(8589):795, 1988.

Raasch B, Maclennan R, Wronski I, Robertson I: Body site specific incidence of basal and squamous cell carcinoma in an exposed population, Townsville, Australia. *Mutat Res* 422:101, 1998.

Ramani ML, Bennett RG: High prevalence of skin cancer in World War II servicemen stationed in the Pacific theater. *J Am Acad Dermatol* 28:733, 1993.

Roth JJ, Granick MS: Squamous cell carcinoma and adnexal carcinomas of the skin. *Clin Plast Surg* 24:687, 1997.

Rowe DE, Carroll RJ, Day CL: Long-term recurrence rates in previously untreated (primary) basal cell carcinoma: Implications for patient follow-up. *J Dermatol Surg Oncol* 15:315, 1989.

Schwartz RA: The actinic keratosis: A perspective and update. *Dermatol Surg* 23:1009, 1997.

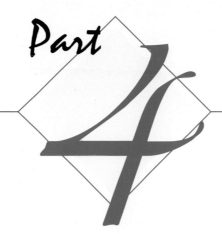

Part 4

Miscellaneous
Skin Diseases

Alopecia

Background

Hair loss, or alopecia, is a common affliction of both men and women. In addition to the obvious cosmetic impact of hair loss, it may have significant psychosocial consequences. Although there are numerous potential etiologies of hair loss, this chapter concentrates on three of the more commonly encountered forms: androgenetic alopecia (AGA), alopecia areata (AA), and telogen effluvium (TE).

Androgenetic alopecia, also known as common baldness, male-pattern baldness, and female-pattern baldness, is an inherited androgen-dependent form of hair loss. Although it affects both men and women, men usually experience more severe hair loss. Alopecia areata, which is felt to be an autoimmune disease, represents a potentially reversible, patchy form of hair loss that may occur on any hair-bearing area of the body. It may present as anything from small, circular areas of hair loss on the scalp to total body hair loss. Telogen effluvium represents a shift of more hairs into the telogen (resting) phase of the hair cycle, with resultant shedding of these normal hairs. Multiple factors, including hormones, nutrition, medications, and systemic disease, are known to incite this condition.

Basic Hair Biology

To understand the pathophysiology of disease states of the hair, one must have a basic understanding of normal hair physiology. Hairs may be divided into terminal and vellus hairs. Terminal hairs are the longer, thicker, more deeply pigmented hairs found on the scalp and eyebrows. The follicles of terminal hair generally extend all the way down into the subcutaneous fat during their growth phase. Vellus hairs are the smaller downy hairs that cover the remainder of the body except the palms and soles. The follicles of vellus hairs are shorter as well as thinner and do not extend deeper than the dermis. All hairs go through three phases during their development (Fig. 18-1). Anagen is the growth phase of the cycle and, although it varies from person to person, generally is thought to last about 3 years for the terminal hairs of the scalp. Catagen occurs next and is the stage of acute follicular regression during which the follicle is shortened in length and reduced in volume. This stage lasts only approximately 3 weeks. The next stage, known as telogen, is the "resting" phase of the hair cycle. This stage generally lasts 3 months and eventuates in the shedding of a normal hair. Most follicles probably reenter the anagen phase before the hair is shed. These hairs account for the 100 hairs normally lost by the scalp in a given day. In a normal scalp, approximately 90 percent of the hairs are in the anagen phase and 10 percent are in the telogen phase at a given time.

Hair Diseases

Androgenetic Alopecia

PATHOPHYSIOLOGY

Androgenetic alopecia is believed to be inherited in an autosomal dominant pattern with incomplete penetrance. Although it is known to occur in all races, its

Figure 18-1

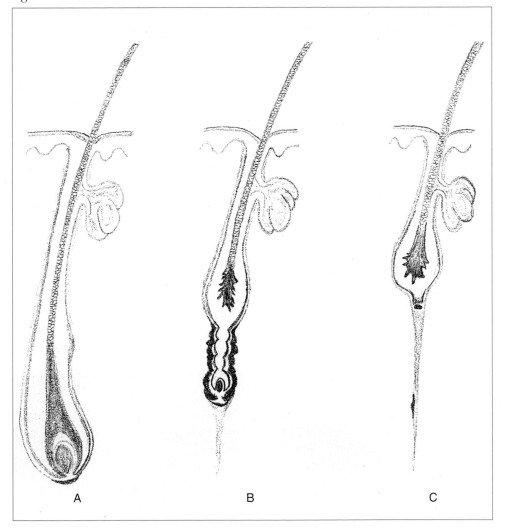

Diagrammatic representation of the phases of the hair growth cycle. *A.* Anagen. *B.* Catagen. *C.* Telogen.

prevalence in whites may approach 100 percent in individuals who reach old age. AGA occurs as a result of transformation of terminal hair follicles into more vellus-like hair follicles. This occurs as a slow process, with each follicular cycle resulting in a hair of shorter length and decreased diameter. The cause of this process was assumed to be endogenous androgens such as testosterone, but this hypothesis is difficult to reconcile with the fact that androgens result in terminal hair differentiation in other parts of the body (axilla, chest, beard) at puberty. It now is felt that AGA probably results from local differences on the scalp in the amounts of enzymes that convert weak androgens such as dehydroepiandrosterone (DHEA) into more potent androgens such as testosterone and dihydrotestosterone. Two of these enzymes are 5α-reductase and aromatase.

CLINICAL PRESENTATION

Androgenetic alopecia may present as early as the late teens in some patients. These patients may complain of thinning hair, a receding hairline, or increased hair on a comb or brush or in the shower. There often is a positive family history for AGA. On examination, men most often initially demonstrate bitemporal recession of the hairline. Over time, the frontal hairline continues to recede, with subsequent thinning of the hair over the vertex of the scalp Figs. 18-2 and 18-3). In women, the frontal hairline is maintained with diffuse hair loss that is somewhat accentuated at the crown. Women who demonstrate deep frontotemporal recession as is seen in men, especially in the presence of hirsutism, acne, and menstrual cycle irregularities, should be evaluated for a hyperandrogen state such as polycystic ovary syndrome. Women frequently develop AGA in the fifth and sixth decades, after the menopause period. No loss of follicles (follicular dropout) is seen, as in "scarring alopecias" such as lichen planopilaris and follicular degeneration syndrome. Instead, there is replacement of the long thick terminal hairs by fine vellus hairs.

Early in the process, when the thinning may not be as apparent, creating a part over the frontal or vertex area and comparing the part width with an area on the

Figure 18-2

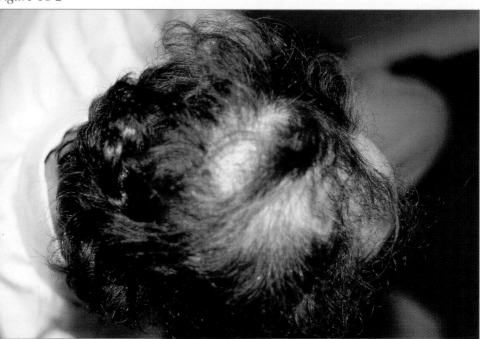

Androgenetic alopecia with diffuse frontal and vertex thinning.

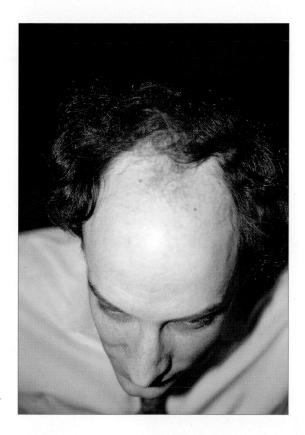

Figure 18-3

Androgenetic alopecia with severe bitemporal recession.

posterior scalp may demonstrate subtle thinning. A hair pull test should be performed by firmly grasping 25 to 30 hairs between the thumb and forefinger and then doing a pull that should cause mild discomfort for the patient. This test on a normal scalp should yield fewer than five normal club hairs. Several pulls on different areas of the scalp should be performed. Early in AGA, when the hair thinning is mild and the hair pull test is diffusely positive, it may be virtually impossible to differentiate AGA from TE.

EVALUATION

Beyond a history and a physical examination, few tests are required. If the history and physical examination fail to yield a definitive diagnosis, the clinician could consider referring this patient to a dermatologist or obtaining a biopsy specimen of the scalp for histologic examination. For all hair conditions, clinicians should instruct the pathologist to section the specimen horizonatally from the epidermis toward the dermis rather than taking the usual vertical approach. This process will show the status of the largest numbers of hair follicles. Other laboratory evaluations are chosen on the basis of the suspected diagnosis.

In women who demonstrate signs of virilization such as severe acne and hirsutism, the evaluation may include free and total testosterone, DHEA sulfate, and sex hormone–binding globulin. If a history of irregular menstrual cycles is present, serum follicle-stimulating hormone (FSH), luteinizing hormone (LH), and serum prolactin levels should be obtained. Adrenal and other tumors may secrete high levels of androgenic hormones. Clinicians should consider further evaluation in select patients.

TREATMENT (FIG. 18-4)

OVERVIEW   Many patients need adequate counseling to understand that AGA is a normal process in both men and women. Societal norms often do not allow this consideration in women, and for many patients of both sexes the loss of hair can be accompanied by a loss of self-confidence, with devastating psychological consequences. Surgical treatments represent the optimal long-term approach. Nevertheless, few patients are ready to commit $10,000 to $20,000 for the mulitple sugical sessions that are required. Topical and systemic therapies are now available that are less expensive over the short term and give patients time to decide about treatment options. Unproven hair growth remedies, the modern equivalent of snake oil, are no more likely to be active than is placebo. Such unproven remedies include ManTop Herbal Hair Tonic, Nature's Hair +, Hair Back, and Fabao 101D.

Figure 18-4

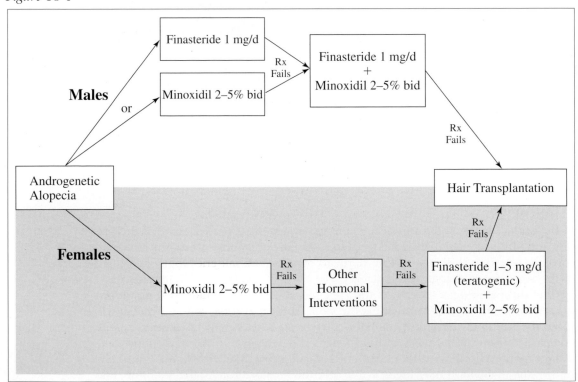

Clinicians should always be cognizant of the powerful effect placebos may have in modern medicine.

We suggest topical minoxidil as the first-line treatment in women and oral finasteride as the first-line treatment in men. When such approaches fail, combination treatment can be initiated, or the patient should be referred for further evaluation. Hormonal approaches beyond finasteride may be used in female patients as an adjunct to other treatment. Hair restoration surgery generally is recommended when patients have not responded to appropriate medical therapy.

SURGERY   Hair restoration surgery has been employed since the 1950s and has undergone a great deal of evolution since that time. A variety of surgical options are available, including hair micrografts, scalp reduction, and scalp lifting. Mini- and micrografting of small groups or individual hair follicles produces the most natural results and is the most expensive and time-consuming approach. This is an excellent but expensive long-term treatment option for many patients. However, not all patients are good candidates for hair restoration surgery. Patients who eventually will lose nearly all their scalp hair, as determined from a consideration of their older relatives' hair loss patterns, are poor candidates. Similarly, patients with a history of poor scar healing may not be good candidates. Patients who express an interest in hair restoration surgery should be referred to a physician with expertise in this area to obtain a consultation regarding surgical options and realistic expectations.

FINASTERIDE   Finasteride is an oral 5α-reductase inhibitor that initially was approved for the treatment of benign prostatic hypertrophy. However, studies have found it to be safe and effective in treating AGA in men at a dose of 1 mg/d. Studies have shown that finasteride statistically significantly increases the numbers of scalp hairs, but increased visual hair density is generally elusive. Whether finasteride can prevent further hair loss for decades is unknown, but it is likely to do so. Although this agent generally is well tolerated, its side effects include erectile dysfunction in about 2 percent of patients. Slowing of hair loss may be seen as early as 3 months into therapy, but hair regrowth usually is not seen until 6 months. If no effect from the medication has been noted after 12 months of therapy, further treatment is unlikely to be beneficial. Once therapy has been initiated, finasteride must be used continually or the hair regrowth that has been attained will be lost. It is uncertain whether men require monitoring of the prostate-specific antigen (PSA) serum level during therapy. Although this is entirely speculative, finasteride theoretically could shrink the prostate and render a prostate tumor less palpable on digital examination. Accordingly, no firm recommendations exist regarding periodic monitoring of PSA.

Use in women is problematic because finasteride may be teratogenic and its efficacy in women is unproven. In postmenopausal women, the teratogenicity of this agent is not relevant. Finasteride may be used in higher doses (2 to 5 mg/d) in women, but controlled studies have not demonstrated the value of this approach.

Finasteride seems to be more effective for inducing hair growth on the vertex of the scalp than in improving temporal recession.

MINOXIDIL   Minoxidil solution was the first drug demonstrated to be safe and effective in growing hair. The patient should apply minoxidil to the scalp twice daily. Patients may not notice any significant regrowth for 3 to 4 months. As with finasteride, increased visual hair density is generally elusive. Whether minoxidil can prevent further hair loss over decades is unknown. Approximately one-third of men experience a modest regrowth, with others achieving stabilization of hair loss. Fewer women than men regrow hair. Like finasteride, minoxidil must be used continually. When the drug is discontinued, the hair that has grown or been retained as a result of minoxidil use falls out 2 to 6 months later. A 2% and a 5% solution of minoxidil are available over the counter. The 5% solution is more efficacious than the lower-strength agent.

MISCELLANEOUS APPROACHES   Anecdotal success has been achieved in some patients by using a combination of oral finasteride and topical minoxidil solution. This combination has not been subjected to clinical evaluation.

Women in the childbearing years with AGA may consider hormonal therapy with oral contraceptives. Oral contraceptives containing progestins with a low androgen index, such as desogestrel (Desogen, Ortho-Cept) and norgestimate (Ortho-Cyclen, Ortho Tri-Cyclen) are preferable. If the AGA is in the early stages, some patients may show improvement in 6 to 12 months. The effect of estrogen replacement after menopause is unproven.

Spironolactone is an older agent that is recommended only occasionally for women with AGA. This potassium-sparing diuretic has been found to decrease testosterone production by the adrenal gland by inhibiting the cytochrome P450 enzyme system. Treatment generally consists of doses of 100 to 200 mg/d and requires monitoring of potassium levels, blood pressure, menstrual changes, and breast tenderness. Before prescribing it, a clinician should carefully review the prescribing information in the *Physician's Desk Reference*.

Alopecia Areata

PATHOPHYSIOLOGY

Alopecia areata (AA) probably is an inflammatory autoimmune condition, although the exact pathophysiology has not been defined. Autoantibodies to anagen hair follicles are present in up to 90 percent of patients with AA. The trigger that initiates the process is unknown. AA affects both sexes equally and is estimated to affect 1 percent of the population by age 50. A positive family history is present in 20 to 30 percent of cases. Although AA has been reported in association with immunologic diseases such as lupus erythematosus, lichen planus, vitiligo, thyroid disease, and pernicious anemia, it is not known whether the occurrence of AA with those conditions occurs by chance or whether other autoimmune processes can foster AA.

CLINICAL PRESENTATION

Alopecia areata most typically presents between 20 and 50 years of age. However, the condition may begin in early childhood and in elderly persons. Patients

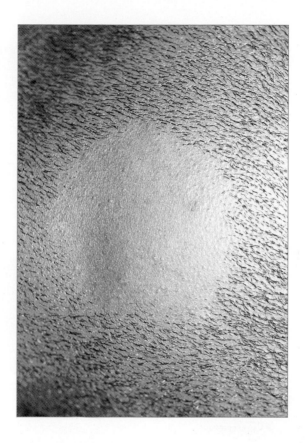

Figure 18-5

Alopecia areata in a young boy.

usually complain of a rather abrupt onset of hair loss that often is localized to one area or only a few specific areas (Figs. 18-5 through 18-8). However, several other patterns of hair loss may be seen in AA, including total scalp hair loss (alopecia totalis), total body hair loss (alopecia universalis), diffuse scalp hair loss (diffuse AA), and localized hair loss along the scalp margin (ophiasis). Although the scalp is the classic site of the disease, other areas, such as the eyebrows and the beard area, may demonstrate hair loss with or without scalp involvement.

The affected areas are nearly devoid of hair. Short "exclamation point" hairs are most prominently seen at the periphery of the alopecia patch. These hairs get their name from their appearance, which is broad at the distal fracture site and then tapers to a smaller diameter more proximally at the scalp. The hair pull test is generally markedly positive at the periphery of the affected area. Nail abnormalities, most frequently pitting of the nails, are seen frequently in patients with AA.

On questioning, some patients may note a tingling, itching, or burning sensation in the area of hair loss. A family history of AA should be obtained as well as a personal history of autoimmune diseases such as vitiligo and thyroid disease. The patient should be questioned about excessive scratching of the scalp or pulling at the hairs in the affected areas to evaluate for possible trichotillomania.

Figure 18-6

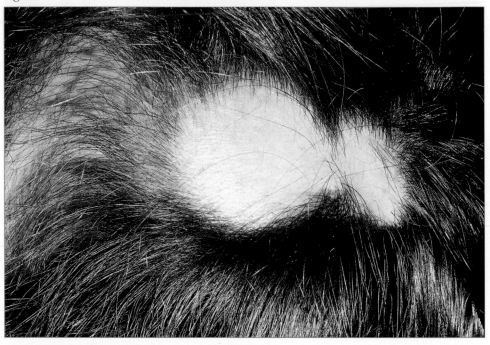

Alopecia areata in an adult.

EVALUATION

If a clinical examination raises suspicion for tinea capitis, one should consider obtaining a specimen for examination by the potassium hydroxide technique and/or obtain a fungal culture. Any evidence of scarring should make clinicians think of other causes of alopecia, including lupus, lichen planus, and other conditions. Serologic testing for thyroid or any other systemic disease has not proved cost-effective.

TREATMENT

Multiple treatment options are available for patients with AA. One useful way of deciding which of the various treatments is appropriate for an individual patient is to decide whether the patient has limited (<50 percent scalp involvement) or extensive (>50 percent scalp involvement) disease.

LIMITED SCALP INVOLVEMENT

No Treatment. "Benign neglect" is rarely advocated. Clinicians should appreciate the fact that hair loss may be psychosocially devastating and that most patients will not accept this approach.

Corticosteroid Agents. For patients with limited involvement of AA, intralesional corticosteroid injection is employed frequently as first-line therapy. Triamcinolone

Figure 18-7

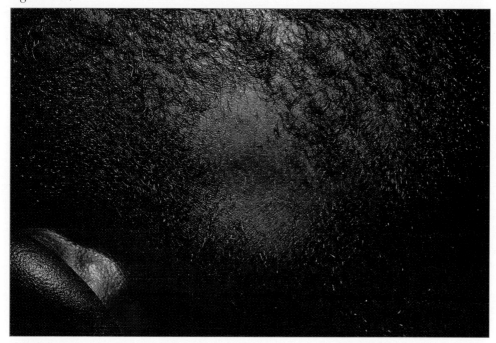

Alopecia areata in a single isolated patch.

acetonide at concentrations from 3 to 10 mg/mL may be injected intradermally into the affected areas as well as into the periphery of the patches. Many clinicians use low concentrations (3 to 5 mg/mL) when large areas of the scalp require injection with as much as 10 mL total volume. Multiple small-volume injections approximately 1 cm apart can be made with a 30-gauge needle. Higher-concentration injections (7.5 to 10 mg/mL) may be used to treat small, isolated patches in patients with limited scalp involvement, and these patients often require only 0.5 to 1.5 mL total volume. Treatments are repeated every 3 to 6 weeks until resolution, and most patients need two to four treatments to bring the disease to resolution. The major potential side effect is atrophy at the injection sites. If sufficient corticosteroid is injected, there is a risk of systemic corticosteroid toxicity.

Topical potent corticosteroid (halobetasol, clobetasol, betamethasone diproprionate, fluocinonide, or a similar agent) application may be effective, particularly if a patient has family help in applying the agent to the affected areas. Daily use of these preparations for several months may be required to see an impact.

Miscellaneous Therapies In patients who are unresponsive to intralesional or topical corticosteroids, topical anthralin therapy may be used. Anthralin at concentrations of 0.25 to 1.0% is applied to affected areas of the scalp. Exposure time should be started at 30 min daily and increased as irritation allows. Patients should be

Figure 18-8

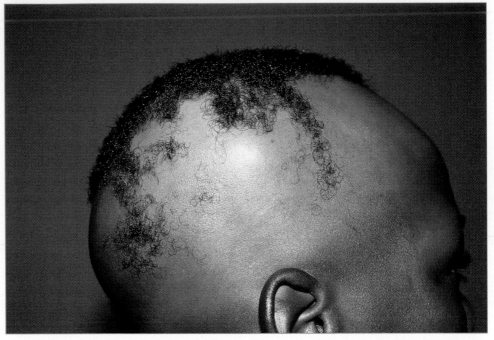

Alopecia areata with severe multicentric loss.

warned to protect treated skin against sun exposure and to be aware of the potential of anthralin to stain clothes and skin.

Another topical therapeutic option is minoxidil solution. There are no data suggesting that this agent is efficacious in AA, but its use is anecdotally advocated. The patient should apply it to the scalp twice daily.

Although most frequently used in patients with extensive AA, topical immunotherapy occasionally may be used in patients with limited AA that is refractory to other treatments. The details of topical immunotherapy are described in the section below.

EXTENSIVE SCALP INVOLVEMENT   For patients with extensive or total scalp involvement, there is no ideal treatment. Many of the treatments used for limited disease may be implemented for patients with more extensive disease, including minoxidil solution, anthralin with or without minoxidil, and superpotent topical corticosteroid plus minoxidil.

A therapeutic modality with anecdotal reports of success is topical immunotherapy. Clinicians apply contact sensitizers such as squaric acid dibutyl ester, dinitrochlorobenzene, and diphencyprone, and the patient becomes sensitized to them. Continued application at concentrations ranging from 0.0001 to 2% then are regularly applied to the scalp to maintain mild erythema. If regrowth is seen, it occurs within 3 months.

Another treatment modality occasionally employed is PUVA therapy. Psoralen (an ultraviolet light photosensitizing agent) administered topically or systemically followed by exposure to ultraviolet A light has had a few anecdotal reports of success.

The use of systemic corticosteroids in this group of patients is controversial, because although these agents are often effective, this is often a chronic disease, and their long-term side effects generally preclude their use. If used at all, they should be used for only a month at a time to gain control of the disease when it is very active. There should be subsequent or concomitant administration of one of the other therapies described above to maintain the therapeutic response.

Telogen Effluvium

PATHOPHYSIOLOGY

Telogen effluvium results from a disturbance of the hair growth cycle that is manifested by the drastically increased loss of normal hairs. Telogen effluvium is seen most commonly in the postpartum period. Other risk factors include discontinuation of birth control pills or high-dose systemic corticosteroids, the use of various medications, high fever, extreme calorie restriction, hypothyroidism, blood loss, and shock. TE is proposed to occur by any of five different mechanisms. Immediate anagen release occurs when some signal causes follicles that normally would complete a longer cycle to enter telogen prematurely. This type of TE often is due to drugs or high fever and is characterized by a short onset (3 to 5 weeks). Delayed anagen release occurs when some signal causes some follicles to remain in a prolonged anagen rather than normally cycling into telogen. When the signal is removed, all these follicles simultaneously cycle into telogen and are shed. This probably represents the form of telogen that occurs in the postpartum period, generally 3 to 4 months after giving birth.

The short-anagen form of telogen effluvium occurs when a chronically shortened anagen phase leads to a higher proportion of follicles being in telogen at any given time. These patients experience a persistent telogen effluvium and the inability to grow long hair. An immediate telogen release type of TE occurs when some signal leads to shortening of the normal telogen phase and immediate entry into anagen. Drugs are felt to be the cause of this type of TE, which is characterized by a relatively short onset. Delayed telogen release is felt to occur when a signal that has led to a longer period of telogen and a subsequent higher proportion of hairs in telogen is released. This is felt to account for the uncommonly observed phenomenon in which relatively mild TE occurs in individuals traveling from low-daylight to high-daylight conditions.

CLINICAL PRESENTATION

Patients generally complain of increased loss of hair when brushing the hair or showering. They may or may not note a significant thinning of the hair. The onset of TE is more abrupt than that of AGA, and patients notice hairs coming out by the handful. TE can be difficult to recognize or assess by physical examination.

The evaluation of overall hair density by inspection is often of little help, as hair density may need to be as much as 50 percent reduced before becoming clinically apparent. However, if thinning is noticeable, it is generally of a diffuse nature. A hair pull test that is positive in multiple areas of the scalp is very suggestive of TE, but a negative test does not exclude the diagnosis because the effluvium may have ended and be in a state of resolution.

Patients have to be asked specific and detailed questions about the predisposing factors. A detailed medical history is required and should include a history of recent pregnancy, recent initiation of or discontinuation of birth control pills, a drug history that includes prescription and nonprescription drugs, recent extreme dieting or weight loss, recent high fever or serious illness, and any symptoms of hypothyroidism. A list of drugs and chemicals that may cause telogen effluvium is shown in Table 18-1.

Table 18-1

Drugs and Chemicals that May Cause Telogen Effluvium

Allopurinol
Androgens (danazol)
Angiotensin-converting enzyme inhibitors (captopril, enalopril)
Anticholesterolemic agents (clofibrate, triparanol)
Anticoagulants (coumarin, dextran, heparin, heparinoids)
Antimitotic agents (colchicine, methotrexate)
Antithyroid medications (carbamazole, methylthiouracil, propylthiourcil)
Benzimidazoles (albendazole, mebendazole)
Beta blockers (systemic: metoprolol, propranolol; topical: betaxalol, levobunolol, timolol)
Bromocriptine
Cimetidine
Gold
Immunoglobulin
Interferon α
Levodopa
Methylsergide
Minoxidil
Oral contraceptives
Proguanil
Psychotropic medications (amphetamines, desipramine, dixyrazine, fluoxetine, imipramine, lithium, transcypromine, valproic acid)
Prostigmine bromide
Retinoids
Sulfasalazine
Terfenadine
Vitamin A

SOURCE: Adapted from Elise A. Olsen, *Disorders of Hair Growth*. New York, McGraw-Hill, 1994, p. 250.

EVALUATION

If an obvious etiology of the TE such as the postpartum period is not evident, further evaluation should include screening for hypothyroidism and iron deficiency.

TREATMENT

The mainstay of treatment is patient education. The patient should be educated about the basics of the hair cycle and why this has occurred. The patient should be reassured that an increase in hair falling out generally precedes hair regrowth but that a great deal of patience is required for a cosmetically acceptable recovery as a hair shaft grows only 0.25 mm/d. Accordingly, patients may require 6 months to note improvement. Occasionally an episode of TE unmasks a previously subclinical AGA, and although hair regrowth will occur, the hair will not regain its previous density.

Possible etiologies that are reversible, such as hypothyroidism, iron deficiency, and extreme dieting, should be corrected. Whenever it is safe to do so, medications that may be causative should be discontinued.

Bibliography

Fiedler VC, Alaiti S: Treatment of alopecia areata. *Dermatol Clin* 14:733, 1996.

Headington JT: Telogen effluvium: New concepts and review. *Arch Dermatol* 129:356, 1993.

Hoffman R, Happle R: Topical immunotherapy in alopecia areata: What, how and why? *Dermatol Clin* 14:739, 1996.

Kaufman KD: Androgen metabolism as it affects hair growth in androgenetic alopecia. *Dermatol Clin* 14:697, 1996.

Pericin M, Trueb RM: Topical immunotherapy of severe alopecia areata with diphenylcyclopropenone: Evaluation of 68 cases. *Dermatology* 196:418, 1998.

Rebora A: Telogen effluvium. *Dermatology* 195:209, 1997.

Rietschel RL: A simplified approach to the diagnosis of alopecia. *Dermatol Clin* 14:691, 1996.

Rokhsar CK, Shupack JL, Vafai JJ, Washenik K: Efficacy of topical sensitizers in the treatment of alopecia areata. *J Am Acad Dermatol* 39:751, 1998.

Rubin MB: Androgenetic alopecia: Battling a losing proposition. *Postgrad Med* 102:129, 1997.

Sawaya ME: Clinical updates in hair. *Dermatol Clin* 15:37, 1997.

Shapiro J: Alopecia Areata: Update on therapy. *Dermatol Clin* 11:35, 1993.

Stough DB, Miner JE: Male pattern alopecia: Surgical options. *Dermatol Clin* 15:609, 1997.

Tobin DJ, Hann SK, Song MS, Bystryn JC: Hair follicle structures targeted by antibodies in patients with alopecia areata. *Arch Dermatol* 133:57, 1997.

Xerosis (Dry Skin)

Background

Xerosis, or dry skin, is seen frequently by clinicians. It is a condition that predisposes patients toward developing dermatitis and pruritus. Although it may be seen in young atopic patients, it becomes more common with advancing age. Moisturizing creams and lotions can penetrate the skin, restore the damaged epidermal barrier, increase epidermal hydration, decrease irritation, and suppress inflammation. Long thought to provide only symptomatic relief for cosmetic conditions, moisturizers are beginning to be viewed as important pharmaceutical agents for medical conditions.

A study of a select group of elderly individuals found that 61 percent thought that they had "dry skin," although xerosis was found in 85 percent. In a study conducted by this author, 60 percent of a community-dwelling elderly population had xerotic skin. Thus, xerosis is exceedingly common.

Risk Factors

Xerosis occurs in association with common inflammatory skin diseases such as atopic dermatitis, in systemic conditions such as hypothyroidism, and as a result of normal human aging (Table 19-1).

Winter weather in cold climates may promote the development of xerosis through increased transepidermal water loss. When the indoor humidity falls relatively low for several consecutive days, the skin is at risk of severe xerosis. Indoor heated environments are seldom humidified adequately.

Pathophysiology

With aging, the skin and its appendages undergo processes that are associated with xerosis. The main alterations that promote xerosis include changes in the number of blood vessels, anatomic changes in the dermoepidermal junction and epidermal cells, and altered function of oil and sweat secretion. The number of minute capillary loops that course through the superficial dermis decreases. This diminished vascularity may be appropriate for an older person's decreased metabolism, but it impedes fluid exchange, wound healing, and heat dissipation. The undulating rete pegs that connect the epidermis to the underlying dermis flatten with age, decreasing the surface area for fluid and nutrient exchange between the dermis and the epidermis. Because of the diminished vascularity and the flattened dermoepidermal junction, the amount of water that passes from the dermis through the epidermis—the transepidermal water loss—decreases. In older epidermis, there is less fluid to be lost.

The epidermal cells also are altered in aging. These cells are larger than their more youthful counterparts and show decreased adhesion. An analogy is that the youthful epidermis works like a brick wall, with mortar firmly attaching each cell. Older skin has irregularity in brick size, and the mortar is cracked and crumbling.

The glands in the skin also show age-related changes. Normally, sweat gland activity pours water onto the skin surface and helps hydrate the skin. However, sweat gland production decreases with age. The sebaceous glands are important because they manufacture natural oils that prevent water loss and lubricate the skin and hairs. It once was thought that sebaceous glands do not function properly in the elderly. However, recent evidence suggests that sebum secretion does not decline with increasing age but that the composition of the sebaceous product differs with aging. Sebum sebaceous wax ester secretion decreases 23 percent

Table 19-1

Causes of Xerosis

Ichthyosis syndromes	Hypervitaminosis A
Ichthyosis vulgaris	Endocrine disorder
Lamellar ichthyosis	Thyroid disease
Nonbullous congentital	Hypoparathyroidism
ichthyosiform erythrodermis	Malignancy
Epidermolytic hyperkeratosis	Carcinoma (lung, cervix, breast,
Multisystem disorders with	leiomyosarcoma, Kaposi's
ichthyosis [e.g., Refsum's	sarcoma)
syndrome, KID (Senter)	Lymphoma (Hodgkin's and mycosis
syndrome, trisomy 21]	fungoides)
Drug-induced	Immune diseases
Hypocholesterolemic agents	Connective tissue disorders
Nicotinic acid	(especially systemic lupus
Triparanol	erythematosus)
Diazocholesterol	Sjögren's syndrome
Clofazamine	Infections and Infestations
Cimetidine	Human immunodefienciency virus
Tretinoin, isotretinoin, and acitretin	Human T-cell lymphotropic virus
Flutamide	type II
Metabolic	Leprosy
Aging	Scabies
Hepatic dysfunction	Miscellaneous causes
Renal failure	Sarcoidosis
Nutritional	Radiotherapy
Malabsorption syndromes	Stasis dermatitis
Kwashiorkor	Venous or arterial insufficiency
Zinc deficiency	Environmental (low humidity
Essential fatty acid deficiency	conditions and cold weather)

SOURCE: Adapted with permission from Golkar and Eichenfield (1998).

per decade after age 35 in men and 32 percent per decade in women. Similarly, there is an alteration in the fatty acid composition in aging sebum compared with the sebum of youth. Thus, sebaceous gland production does not decline, but the product is different. Less water comes to the surface with less sweat, and the natural oil made is not the same.

Xerotic skin predisposes patients toward developing irritant contact dermatitis. A recent study demonstrated that irritant contact dermatitis is less likely to occur on well-moisturized skin compared with xerotic skin. Accordingly, xerosis is a predisposing factor for other skin conditions.

In inflammatory disease such as atopic dermatitis, xerosis indicates subclinical inflammation. Pruritus may be due to skin diseases such as scabies and contact dermatitis and systemic diseases such as hyperthyroidism and malignancy, or it may have idiopathic causes. In hypothyroidism, as in most other systemic conditions, the mechanism by which xerosis is produced remains elusive.

Clinical Presentation

Xerotic skin appears scaly and rough and may have increased lines (Fig. 19-1). Although xerosis is most common on the extremities, it may be seen anywhere on the body. When certain specific body sites are involved, clinicians should suspect other conditions. For instance, a xerotic scalp should make a clinician consider seborrheic dermatitis. Xerotic antecubital and popliteal fossae in a child should raise the possibility of atopic dermatitis.

As was stated above, xerosis can predispose patients toward dermatitis and pruritus. This condition appears as rough, scaly skin with a background or erythema,

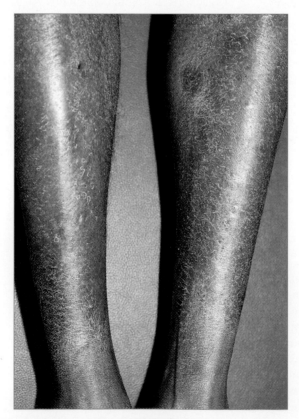

Figure 19-1

Severe xerosis in an elderly patient.

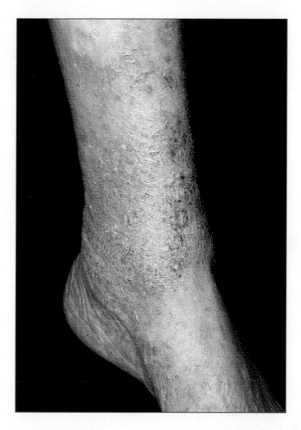

Figure 19-2

Xerotic dermatitis.

possible exudate, and secondary changes that include excoriations and lichenification (Fig. 19-2).

Evaluation

Beyond physical examination, further investigation is warranted only if other conditions are suspected. Chronic unexplained pruritus warrants a careful history, a physical examination, and appropriate tests for systemic conditions (Table 19-2). If a pharmacologic agent is suspected of being a cause of dry skin and can be discontinued safely, patients may benefit from this approach. Dry skin and increased scaliness have been reported with beta blockers; busulfan; clofibrate; nafoxidine; niacin; retinoids such as acitretin, etretinate, and isotretinoin; and tamoxifen.

Table 19-2

Systemic Diseases that May Present as Generalized Itching

Endocrine diseases	Gastrointestinal tract cancers:
Autoimmune progesterone or	tongue, stomach, and colon
estrogen dermatitis	Kaposi's sarcoma
Diabetes mellitus	Leukemia
Perimenopausal itching	Lung cancer
Thyroid disease	Malignant mastocytoma
Hematologic diseases	Multiple myeloma
Hypereosinophilic syndrome	Non-Hodgkin's lymphomas
Iron deficiency	Polycythemia rubra vera
Job's syndrome	Prostatic carcinoma
Paraproteinemia (myelomatosis)	Thyroid carcinoma
Polycythemia vera	Uterine carcinoma
Liver diseases	Neuropsychiatric diseases
Biliary atresia	Focal central nervous system
Carcinoma of pancreatic head or	diseases
bile ducts	Psychiatric conditions and itching
Choledocholithiasis	Psychogenic itching
Cholestasis of pregnancy	Neurotic excoriations
Chronic pancreatitis	Monosymptomatic hypochondriacal
Drug-induced hepatitis and/or	psychosis
cholestasis	Pharmacologic causes
Hemochromatosis	Pregnancy
Hepatitis B and C	Polymorphic eruption of pregnancy
Primary biliary cirrhosis	Herpes gestationis (pemphigoid
Primary sclerosing cholangitis	gestationis)
Malignancy	Pruritic folliculitis of pregnancy
Breast carcinoma	Intrahepatic cholestasis of pregnancy
Carcinoid syndrome	(pruritus gravidarum)
Cutaneous T-cell lymphoma	Renal diseases
Hodgkin's disease	

Therapy

Overview

Patients benefit from hearing recommendations for moisturizer therapy from clinicians. Moisturizers may be used alone or in conjunction with therapeutic ingredients (Fig. 19-3).

Figure 19-3

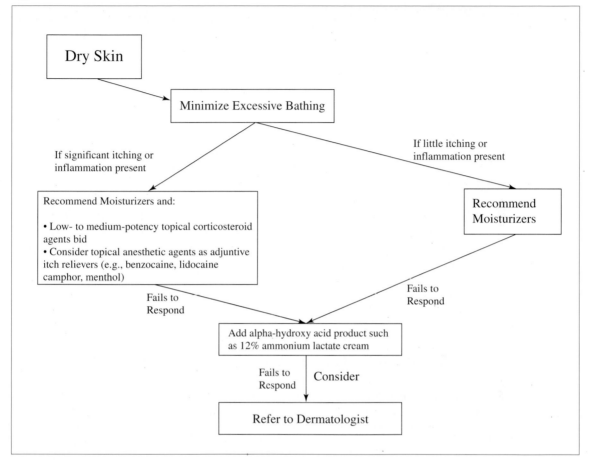

Algorithm for treatment of xerosis.

Scientific Rationale for Using Moisturizers

Moisturizers are an essential component of therapy in present or suspected cases of xerosis. Moisturizers can help the skin in a variety of ways. Xerotic skin has decreased skin extensibility, and hydration clearly improves skin extensibility. Water softens the horny layer and allows a rapid improvement in extensibility, particularly in women and older persons. It is reasonable to assume that if the skin is more extensible, it is less likely to crack or tear. Topical moisturizers increase skin hydration, presumably by trapping water that normally is lost through the skin.

Normally, the skin performs a barrier function to seal in fluids and seal out bacteria and noxious substances. Fatty acids and other lipids are necessary for this epidermal barrier function. Lipids applied to the surface of the skin do not sit on the surface like a layer of plastic wrap; they penetrate throughout the entire stratum corneum between keratinocytes and help restore barrier function.

In augmenting the epidermal barrier, moisturizer preparations provide protection against irritation. Moisturizers also prevent irritant contact dermatitis from excessive detergent exposure. Irrational bathing habits such as the use of scalding hot water and washing head to toe daily with harsh soaps exacerbate xerosis and should be discontinued. These activities remove both natural lipids and the best moisturizers.

Beyond mere protection, topically applied lipids may suppress the oxidation of arachidonic acid, thus decreasing the generation of known chemotactic and proinflammatory substances. The mechanism by which this may occur is unknown, but this process has been demonstrated in laboratory models. Even when topical corticosteroid agents are required for treating inflammatory skin diseases, the addition of moisturizers may decrease the amount required. Moisturizers may even be effective for noninflammatory skin diseases such as the pruritus of liver disease.

In short, moisturizers can penetrate the skin, increase epidermal hydration, decrease irritation, and suppress inflammation. There is a scientifically valid rationale for their use.

Moisturizer Therapy

TERMINOLOGY

Moisturizers add water to the skin, and water is the simplest moisturizer. Because the skin dries rapidly, the hydrating effect of water is lost within several minutes. Therefore, most moisturizers contain a moisturizer to enhance the product's effectiveness. Moisturizers are compounds that contain lipids whose purpose is to seal water into the skin. Water may come from the moisturizer preparation itself or from transepidermal water loss.

OINTMENTS AND OILS

Petrolatum, more widely known as petroleum jelly, is the principal ingredient in many moisturizing ointments. Petrolatum has been studied extensively and may be one of the best moisturizers. Its advantages include that it is inexpensive, occlusive, and substantive. Unfortunately, patients find petrolatum too greasy. It works optimally when applied immediately after bathing to seal in the moisture. Arthritis may limit the ability of some patients to apply such thick ointments. Moisturizer oils such as mineral oil have many of the same benefits as petrolatum. They generally do not last as long but are slightly less greasy and easier to apply.

All pure moisturizer ointments and oils share one problem: They contain no water within them and thus may not last long enough on the skin for complete hydration to occur. This limitation may be partially overcome by applying a moisturizer immediately after bathing, sealing in the acquired moisture.

CREAMS AND LOTIONS

To improve their cosmetic appeal, moisturizer lipids can be whipped with water, color, and fragrance to make creams and lotions. The main difference between creams and lotions is their water content: The more water, the thinner the preparation. Lotions have more water than do creams. Compared with oils and ointments, creams and lotions have better cosmetic appeal because they are more elegant to apply. Some seem to disappear easily into the skin, a characteristic favored by many patients. These cosmetic aspects of moisturizers should not be overlooked, as they can increase patient use and compliance. Additionally, because creams and lotions contain water, it has been shown that oil-in-water emulsions hydrate skin better than does petrolatum alone.

Other ingredients, including alcohols and other solvents, further thin the preparation and stabilize the other ingredients. Lotions and creams generally are composed of an emulsion of oil and water. Typical ingredients include water, mineral oil, propylene glycol, stearic acid, and petrolatum or lanolin. To keep the preparation from separating, most also contain triethanolamine stearate or another emulsifier. Humectants, such as glycerin and sorbitol bind water and may promote stratum corneum hydration. Proteins and collagen may act as humectants, or water-binding agents, but these proteins are too large to penetrate the stratum corneum.

Creams and lotions not only are more effective but also are widely accepted by patients. Preparations such as Moisturel, Lubriderm, and Curèl are free of common sensitizers such as lanolin and fragrance. Although heavily scented products have market appeal to some patients, the authors rarely recommend them because of the potential allergenicity of the fragrances.

THERAPEUTIC INGREDIENTS

TOPICAL COOLING AND SOOTHING PREPARATIONS Many physicians also employ medicated lotions with anesthetics. The advantage of these agents is that they can provide noncorticosteroidal itch relief in the setting of xerosis. Camphor and menthol are anesthetic agents and may be useful for relieving pruritus. Camphor has a potent medical smell that some individuals like and others hate. Menthol provides an immediate cooling sensation. Other widely used anesthetic agents that are relatively safe include benzocaine and lidocaine. The "caine" anesthetics provide effective, rapid relief of itching and burning symptoms. These ingredients may be particularly beneficial in the setting of xerotic dermatitis. The role of these agents is to provide itch relief at the same time moisturization is occurring. If patients can feel therapeutic benefit from a preparation, they may be more likely to use it, and may avoid damaging scratching behavior. Like all additives, these agents may rarely be allergenic in some individuals.

ALPHA-HYDROXY ACIDS Alpha-hydroxy acids such as pyruvic, glycolic, and lactic acids are found in certain fruits, including apples, grapes, and oranges. Despite their wide characterization as "fruit," most commercially available products use synthetic rather than natural sources of these agents. Although there has been a great deal of lay enthusiasm for these compounds, only one of these acids, lactic acid, has been studied extensively.

The commercial form of lactic acid, ammonium lactate, is a prescription preparation that is useful for the treatment of severe xerosis, ichthyosis and their associated itching. Not only does it improve the appearance of skin, controlled trials have demonstrated that it restores the normal desquamative process, increases the thickness of the viable epidermis, and alters the structure of the dermis. In the 12% concentration, ammonium lactate cream (Lac-Hydrin 12%) has been found effective in vehicle-controlled studies in decreasing moderate to severe xerosis. Additionally, the keratolytic effect can be helpful in restoring the normal thickness of the skin to thick cracked soles. Ammonium lactate preparations are more effective than are ordinary moisturizers such as Eucerin.

Clinicians should note that cosmetic and other product manufacturers are required to state the ingredients that have been added, not the ingredients present in the final product. Careful scrutiny of labels will reveal sodium hydroxide as a common over-the-counter ingredient in acid products. As a result, many over-the-counter alpha-hydroxy acid products contain little or no bioavailable acid. Ammonium lactate in the form of Lac-Hydrin 12% cream has been found to be more efficacious than alpha-hydroxy acid products such as Lacticare.

UREA　Urea has been found to have therapeutic activity in hydrating the skin. Concentrations of 3 to 10% may increase epidermal hydration better than does the moisturizer vehicle alone. Although few controlled studies have been performed with this agent, further work may reveal the value of urea in promoting cutaneous hydration.

TOPICAL CORTICOSTEROID AGENTS　In the setting of significant visible inflammation, topical corticosteroid agents may be used in adddition to moisturizers to decrease such inflammation quickly. Mild disease may respond to hydrocortisone or similar weak topical agents, whereas more marked inflammation may require more potent agents.

Summary

Xerosis and its common result pruritus occur frequently in the population. Xerosis is not due to decreased lipid production. Instead, there is a decrease in dermal vascularity and sweat secretion, and there are structural alterations in the dermoepidermal junction and epidermal cells. The types of lipids produced by oil glands change, but the quantity does not decrease. Moisturizer ointments, creams, and lotions can penetrate the skin, increase epidermal hydration, decrease irritancy, and suppress inflammation. Extensive research suggests that moisturizers should be viewed as important pharmaceutical agents for treating medical conditions. Therapeutic ingredients such as menthol, alpha-hydroxy acids, and urea may offer benefit beyond routine moisturizer therapy. By educating their patients, clinicians can help develop strategies for the relief of xerosis and pruritus.

Bibliography

Beauregard S, Gilchrest BA: A survey of skin problems and skin care regimens in the elderly. *Arch Dermatol* 123:1638, 1987.

Downing DT, Stewart ME, Strauss JS: Changes in sebum secretion and the sebaceous gland. *Dermatol Clin* 4:419, 1986.

Draelos ZK: *Cosmetics in Dermatology.* Churchill Livingstone, 1990.

Fenske NA, Lober CW: Skin changes of aging: Pathological implications. *Geriatrics* 45(3):27, 1990.

Fleischer AB Jr: Pruritus in the elderly: Management by senior dermatologists. *J Am Acad Dermatol* 28(4):603, 1993.

Ghiadially R, Halkier-Sorensen L, Elias PM: Effects of petrolatum on stratum corneum structure and function. *J Am Acad Dermatol* 26:387, 1992.

Gilchrest BA: *Skin and Aging Processes.* Boca Raton, CRC Press, 1984.

Golkar L, Eichenfield LF. Xerosis and systemic disease: Are you undertreating your dry skin patients? *Skin Aging* 6:35, 1998.

Hannuksela A, Kinnunen T: Moisturizers prevent irritant dermatitis. *Acta Dermatoveneriol* 72:42, 1992.

Jacobsen E, Billings JK, Frantz RA, et al: Age-related changes in sebaceous wax ester secretion rates in men and women. *J Invest Dermatol* 85:483, 1985.

Loden M: The increase in skin hydration after application of emollients with different amounts of lipids. *Acta Dermatovenereol* 72(5):327, 1992.

Rogers RS, Callen J, Wehr R, Krochmal L: Comparative efficacy of 12% ammonium lactate lotion and 5% lactic acid lotion in the treatment of moderate to severe xerosis. *J Am Acad Dermatol* 21:714, 1989.

Thorne EG: Coping with pruritus: A common geriatric complaint. *Geriatrics* 33:47, 1978.

Watsky KL, Freije L, Leneveu MC, et al: Water-in-oil emollients as steroid sparing adjunctive therapy in the treatment of psoriasis. *Cutis* 50:383, 1992.

Wehr R, Kantor I, Jones EL, et al: A controlled comparative efficacy study of 5% ammonium lactate lotion versus an emollient control lotion in the treatment of moderate xerosis. *J Am Acad Dermatol* 25:849, 1991.

Wehr RF, Krochmal L: Considerations in selecting a moisturizer. *Cutis* 39:512, 1987.

Wehr R, Krochmal L, Bagatell F, Ragsdale W: A controlled two-center study of lactate 12 percent lotion and a petrolatum-based creme in patients with xerosis. *Cutis* 37;205, 1986.

Wilhelm K-P, Cua AB, Maibach HI: Skin aging: Effect on transepidermal water loss, stratum corneum hydration, skin surface pH and casual sebum content. *Arch Dermatol* 127:1806, 1991.

Yamamoto A, Serizawa S, Ito M, Sato Y: Effect of aging on sebaceous gland activity on the fatty acid composition of wax esters. *J Invest Dermatol* 89:507, 1987.

Vitiligo

Background

Vitiligo is a common acquired depigmenting disorder that is characterized by well-demarcated patches of depigmented skin. The cutaneous depigmentation results from the loss of melanocytes in the affected areas. Vitiligo affects approximately 1 to 3 percent of the population, usually presents by age 40, and shows no racial, sexual, or regional differences.

Etiology

The depigmented lesions of vitiligo are caused by the loss of melanocytes in the skin. The cause of this loss is not known. The three major and potentially overlapping theories that account for vitiligo are (1) intrinsic melanocyte dysfunction leading to cell death, (2) autoimmune-mediated cell destruction, and (3) neurochemical compounds released from nerve endings that have a toxic effect on melanocytes. It seems likely that the bulk of melanocyte destruction in vitiligo is due to the second mechanism: autoimmune destruction. Autoantibodies directed against melanocyte antigens are often present in patients' sera, and the inflammatory response in depigmented skin is muted. Supporting the autoimmune theory is the association of other autoimmune diseases with vitiligo. The most frequently associated diseases include thyroid disease, diabetes mellitus, Addison's disease, pernicious anemia, and multiple endocrinopathy syndrome. Given the frequency of vitiligo in the population, many of these reported associations appear to occur purely by chance. Thyroid disease may be an exception, and any sign of thyroid disease should prompt investigation. Congenital nevi may be found more commonly in patients with vitiligo than in the normal population.

Not all melanocytes are lost uniformly in vitiligo. Melanocytes in periorificial areas (around the mouth, eyes, and genital orifices) are more likely to be lost than are other melanocytes. Also, the interfollicular melanocytes are lost in vitiligo, but the melanocytes of the hair bulb (follicular melanocytes) are less likely to be affected. The latter fact is important in cutaneous repigmentation, in which the hair follicle melanocytes serve as the reservoir for repopulating the skin. Therefore, patches of vitiligo on non-hair-bearing skin or skin where the hairs are also depigmented are more resistant to treatment.

There seems to be a genetic component predisposing a person to the development of vitiligo. In some studies, up to 30 percent of patients reported vitiligo in other family members. However, the inheritance pattern does not follow simple Mendelian genetics and probably involves multiple genetic loci.

In addition, certain precipitating factors are noted by many patients. The onset of vitiligo often is attributed to a major emotional stress or severe illness. A significant number of patients also develop lesions of vitiligo at sites of injury or trauma. Exacerbation of disease at sites of trauma is known as Koebner's phenomenon; this phenomenon also occurs in psoriasis and lichen planus.

Clinical Presentation

The typical patient presents between ages 10 and 30 years, concerned about the new appearance of white patches on his or her body. The patient may give a history of the patch or patches remaining stable. More likely, a slow or even rapidly progressive course of depigmentation is reported. The lesions of vitiligo are usually asymptomatic, although patients may complain of being prone to sunburn in affected areas.

The lesions of vitiligo are depigmented, milky white macules or patches 1 to 3 cm in size. The borders of the lesions are usually quite distinct. Often they are distributed on the body in a strikingly symmetric manner, with initial lesions seen commonly on the hands, feet, forearms, anogenital area, face, and lips (Figs. 20-1

Figure 20-1

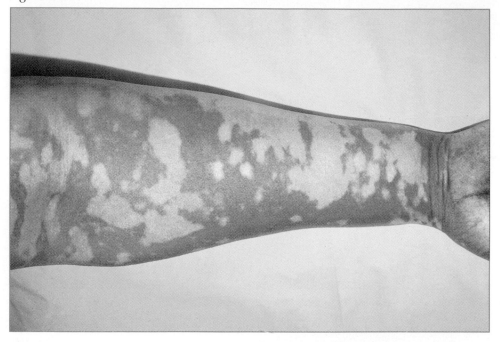

Depigmentation with vitiligo may be so extensive that it may be unclear that the normal skin has the darker color.

through 20-4). As was noted above, vitiligo often demonstrates Koebner's phenomenon in that lesions frequently appear at sites of injury or trauma. The depigmented macules are more clinically apparent on dark-skinned individuals and in sun-exposed areas of lighter-skinned people. In fair-skinned individuals, a Wood's lamp examination may be necessary to detect hypopigmented or depigmented patches; the small amount of pigment in normal fair skin is sufficient to absorb the long ultraviolet (UV) light of the Wood's lamp, increasing the contrast between pigmented and depigmented skin.

The hairs within the macules frequently remain normally pigmented, but in more advanced disease they may be depigmented. Trichrome lesions may be found that demonstrate a band of hypopigmented skin between the completely depigmented central portion of the lesion and the surrounding normally pigmented skin. Occasionally inflamed borders surrounding depigmented lesions are seen; this finding may indicate an early or evolving lesion that may be more responsive to treatment with topical corticosteroids (see below). In addition to the cutaneous manifestations, an ophthalmologic examination may demonstrate pigmentary changes in choroid and retinal pigment or uveitis.

Vitiligo may be subclassified in accordance with the distribution of the lesions. Generalized vitiligo, the most common form, is characterized by varying numbers of widespread macules distributed in a bilateral, symmetric pattern. *Universal*

Figure 20-2

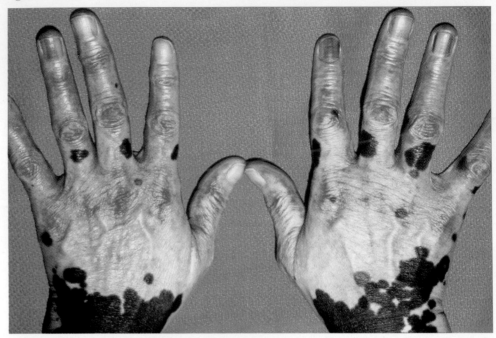

Bilateral symmetry is common in vitiligo.

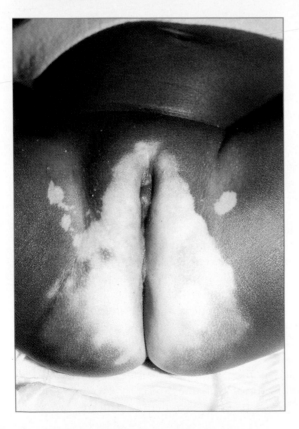

Figure 20-3

Anogenital involvement is common.

Figure 20-4

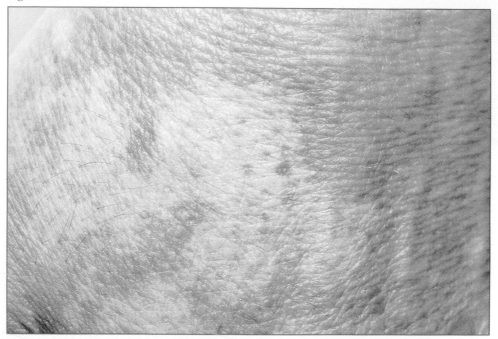

In more lightly pigmented patients, the difference between normal and depigmented skin is more difficult to discern. Sunscreen application to the normal skin minimizes tanning and may help reduce the contrast between affected and unaffected skin.

vitiligo is the term used when this process leaves only a few remaining normal areas of pigmentation. *Acrofacial vitiligo* involves the distal extremities and periorificial facial areas. *Focal or localized vitiligo* describes an isolated macule or a few macules in a discrete area. *Segmental vitiligo* indicates a situation in which the depigmented macules are localized unilaterally to one area of the body, such as a single extremity.

The clinical course of vitiligo is variable. Some patients have limited disease that is stable; others have progressive disease. The extent of disease may change suddenly. Spontaneous resolution may occur, though not commonly.

Evaluation

The diagnosis of vitiligo generally is based on the clinical findings of depigmented macules in a roughly bilaterally symmetric distribution (Table 20-1). A biopsy specimen occasionally is required to confirm the diagnosis and distinguish vitiligo from

Table 20-1

Common Forms of Hypopigmentation

CONDITION	CLINICAL APPEARANCE	MECHANISM
Vitiligo	Depigmented macules in a roughly bilaterally symmetric distribution; can occur in a zosteriform distribution (segmental vitiligo)	Most likely autoimmune-mediated destruction of melanocytes
Piebaldism	White forelock and patch of depigmentation, usually in anterior midline; present at birth	Defect in melanocyte migration during development
Albinism	Many varieties; characterized by decreased to absent pigmentation of all or nearly all skin	Melanocytes are present, but there is a defect in melanin production
Lupus erythematosus	Depigmentation associated with erythema, scarring, "cigarette paper" wrinkling of skin surface; common with hyperpigmentation around depigmented areas	Autoimmune inflammation of skin with destruction of basal layer of epidermis
Sclerodema	Spotty depigmentation of trunk can occur suddenly	Autoimmune-mediated; this type of pigmentary change is associated with systemic sclerosis variant
Idiopathic guttate hypomelanosis	Scattered small white spots on extremities	Benign process; unknown etiology

other diseases that may be depigmenting, such as lupus erythematosus, sarcoidosis, and mycosis fungoides. The specimen should be taken from the border of a lesion. Special stains for melanin or immunohistochemical stains for melanocytes may be used to demonstrate the lack of melanocytes in lesional skin when one is trying to distinguish vitiligo from postinflammatory hypopigmentation. Additional laboratory tests are necessary only when the patient's history or physical examination suggests the presence of another autoimmune disease, such as autoimmune thyroid disease; antimelanocyte antibody tests are done in some research situations but not for diagnostic purposes.

Treatment

General Approaches

While vitiligo is a disease that is only "skin deep," treatment is important because vitiligo can have an extreme psychosocial impact. Vitiligo affects lives in a variety of ways because of social stigmatization, resulting in avoidance of activities and negative reactions by others. Studies have demonstrated an inability of these patients to function up to their potential in school or work because of social rejection. Supportive care should be offered by the clinician, and some patients should be offered a referral to a psychologist or psychiatrist.

Regardless of the form of medical therapy the patient undergoes, it is important that both the physician and the patient have realistic expectations. Any of the repigmenting modalities will take several months to attain optimal results. Both the patient and the physician should be patient and not discard a therapy as a failure until it has been given a 3- to 6-month trial (Table 20-2). The patient should be aware that initial repigmentation occurs around the hair follicle and will give the affected area a speckled appearance. Although a significant improvement may be seen with therapy, treatment is frequently unsatisfactory. Fortunately, in patients who do respond to therapy, maximal repigmentation seems to occur on the face and neck.

It is important that patients be informed that affected areas of their skin are more susceptible to photodamage, including sunburn, and the potential development of skin cancers. The use of sunscreens on lesional skin should be stressed to protect the affected depigmented skin from photoaging. In addition, for patients with fair skin, sunscreens minimize tanning and therefore minimize the contrast between affected and uninvolved skin.

Topical Corticosteroid Agents

Topical corticosteroid therapy is one of the first-line treatment options. This may be due as much to its ease of use and side effect profile as to the clinical efficacy of these products. Midpotency corticosteroids (e.g., triamcinolone, hydrocortisone valerate, fluticasone) applied twice daily should be the initial therapy in young children, while older children and adults may be started on a high-potency corticosteroid (e.g., halobetasol, clobetasol, or betamethasone diproporionate in an optimized vehicle) for the first month or two and then tapered to a lower-potency formulation once a response is noted. The likelihood of success is not known, though it appears to be higher for those with lesions of recent onset and lesions that have signs of active inflammation (redness).

The extensive use of topical corticosteroids can place a patient at risk for hypothalamic-pituitary-adrenal axis suppression. Potent topical corticosteroid agents

Table 20-2

Treatment of Vitiligo

TREATMENT	ADVANTAGES	DISADVANTAGES	BEST CLINICAL SITUATION
Sunscreen	Protects against sunburn; may help limit pigmentation of unaffected skin	Does not affect pigmentation	To prevent burns in fair-skinned patients
Topical corticosteroids	Easy to apply	Limited efficacy; corticosteroid side effects	Limited localized active* disease
Cosmetic coverage	Very effective cosmetically; widely available at department stores	Does not improve pigmentation	Limited or extensive disease
Psoralen with ultraviolet A	Most effective way to repopulate skin with melanocytes	Expensive, time-consuming, acute (burns) and chronic (skin cancer) side effects; repigmentation may be irregular	Highly motivated patient with facial and hand involvement
Surgical techniques	Repopulates melanocytes	Expensive; not available in many areas; repigmentation may be irregular	Localized area with "stable"† disease
Micropigmentation (tattooing)	Permanent	Difficult to match normal skin	Limited involvement of lips
Depigmentation of normal skin	Can give patients one even (depigmented) color; permanent	Permanent	Dark-skinned patients with very extensive vitiligo

* Active disease refers to progressive disease or areas with signs of inflammation (redness).
† Stable disease indicates disease that is nonprogressive and does not have signs of active inflammation.

should be used judiciously, generally limited to 4 to 8 weeks. When using potent topical corticosteroid agents, clinicians should try to use the smallest amount that results in a good response. Potent topical corticosteroids generally should not be used on the face or in intertriginous areas. Adrenal suppression has been demonstrated with as little as 2 g/d of potent agents. When large areas are treated, it may be best not to use a topical corticosteroid stronger than 0.1% triamcinolone cream. Oral corticosteroids generally are not used because of the need for prolonged treatment and the severity of side effects with the long-term use of systemic corticosteroids.

Camouflage Techniques

Patients often benefit from the use of cosmetic camouflage to mask vitiligo lesions. Examples include various brands of makeup, such as Covermark, Dermablend, Derma Color, and Dermage. These cosmetics can be extremely effective at hiding the presence of vitiligo even in patients with normally very dark skin. Alternatively, topical dyes such as Dyoderm, and Vitadye require less frequent application and are more resistant to external forces. These products are most beneficial for use on the face, where the lesions are most visible and the camouflage is less likely to be rubbed off. These products are more easily employed by women than by men because women are more likely to have experience in cosmetic application and because the appearance of foundation on women is an expected societal norm.

In more fair-skinned individuals, the use of dihydroxyacetone-containing instant tanning preparations can offer adequate masking. Great care must be take to avoid darkening the appearance of normal skin.

Phototherapy

Psoralen photochemotherapy (PUVA) generally is considered the most efficacious treatment for increasing the pigment in lesions of vitiligo. It involves administering psoralen to the patient either orally or topically and then exposing the patient to ultraviolet A (UVA) light (320 to 400 nm), which often leads to subsequent repigmentation. The exact mechanism of action of this treatment for vitiligo is unknown. The patient should be prepared to undergo two to three treatments per week for 4 to 12 months. This type of regimen is frequently impractical for patients and requires a highly motivated patient to maintain compliance. Topical PUVA should be considered for patients with involvement of <20 percent of body surface and for children older than 5 years with localized patches of vitiligo. Conversely, oral PUVA may be used in patients with more than 20 percent involvement of the body and those who are recalcitrant to topical PUVA. It is not recommended for children under age 12. Although 70 to 80 percent of patients note some induction of pigment after oral PUVA therapy, less than 20 percent have total repigmentation.

Patients should be counseled about the potential side effects of PUVA therapy, including nausea and vomiting from the use of oral psoralens and the increased risk for the subsequent development of nonmelanoma skin cancers (there also may be some increased risk of melanoma). The risk of skin cancer increases with the number of PUVA treatments. The authors do not use PUVA except in instances in which the phototherapy is administered in the physician's office. Serious burns and death may occur from overexposure to PUVA.

Narrow-band ultraviolet B (UVB) has been found to be as effective as topical PUVA and is thought to have fewer adverse effects (though long-term comparative data are not available). Whether this is also true for standard UVB treatments is not known.

Topical Depigmentation

For patients with more than 50 percent cutaneous depigmentation who have demonstrated therapeutic resistance to the therapies listed above, depigmentation can be considered. Depigmentation is accomplished with the topical application of monobenzylether of hydroquinone (Benoquin). Depigmentation is not a process that should be taken lightly by the patient. This process should be considered permanent and irreversible (as the melanocytes are destroyed) and may take from 6 months to 2 years to complete. This treatment produces albino-like skin tones. Patients and clinicians should realize that depigmentation may occur in areas distant from the application sites.

Surgical Therapies

In addition to the medical therapies described above, a variety of surgical techniques have been developed to transplant melanocytes from unaffected skin to areas of depigmented skin. Autologous skin grafts are multiple small (2 mm) punch grafts taken from unaffected donor sites such as the buttocks and inner arms and transplanted to affected areas. If grafting of a large area is planned, it is advisable to place a limited number of grafts in a small test site to determine the outcome. Spreading of pigment may be seen as early as 4 to 6 weeks after grafting. The repigmented skin may have a cobblestone surface or spotty repigmentation.

Epidermal grafts obtained by suction blisters are another option with less chance of scarring than punch grafts. Epidermis is removed from the recipient site by suction blister, freezing with liquid nitrogen, or dermabrasion before graft placement. Again, incomplete or spotty repigmentation may result.

Micropigmentation (tattooing) involves injecting colored pigments, most commonly iron oxide, into the dermis. This may be most useful in the lip area, particularly for those with dark skin. Unfortunately, many patients experience significant pigment loss within the first several weeks after the procedure. Also, it is quite difficult to obtain a perfect match of pigment with the surrounding skin.

Bibliography

Antoniou C, Katsambas A: Guidelines for the treatment of vitiligo. *Drugs* 43:490, 1992.

Baharav E, Merimski O, Shoenfeld Y, et al: Tyrosinase as an autoantigen in patients with vitiligo. *Clin Exp Immunol* 105:84, 1996.

Boersma BR, Westerhof W, Bos JD: Repigmentation in vitiligo vulgaris by autologous minigrafting: Results in nineteen patients. *J Am Acad Dermatol* 33:990, 1995.

Grimes PE: Vitiligo: An overview of therapeutic approaches. *Dermatol Clin* 11:325, 1993.

Hann SK, Chun WH, Park YK: Clinical characteristics of progressive vitiligo. *Int J Dermatol* 36:353, 1997.

Kent G, Al'Abadie M: Psychologic effects of vitiligo: A critical incident analysis. *J Am Acad Dermatol* 35:895, 1996.

Kovacs SO: Vitiligo. *J Am Acad Dermatol* 38:647, 1998.

Le Poole C, Boissy RE: Vitiligo. *Semin Cutan Med Surg* 16:3, 1997.

Nordlund JJ, Halder RM, Grimes PE: Management of vitiligo. *Dermatol Clin* 11:27, 1993.

Nordlund JJ, Majumder PP: Recent investigations on vitiligo vulgaris. *Dermatol Clin* 15:69, 1997.

Olsson MJ, Juhlin L: Epidermal sheet grafts for repigmentation of vitiligo and piebaldism, with a review of surgical techniques. *Acta Dermatovenereol* 77:463, 1997.

Schallreuter KU, Lemke R, Brandt O, et al: Vitiligo and other diseases: Coexistence or true association? Hamburg study on 321 patients. *Dermatology* 188:269, 1994.

Schwartz RA, Janniger CK: Vitiligo. *Cutis* 60:239, 1997.

Westerhof W, Nieuweboer-Krobotova L: Treatment of vitiligo with UV-B radiation vs topical psoralen plus UV-A. *Arch Dermatol* 133:1525, 1997.

Index

Page numbers followed by an *f* indicate figures; numbers followed by a *t* indicate tables.

ISBN 0-07-022067-0

90000

9 780070 220676